W0037562

Mental Health in Historical Perspective

Series Editors
Catharine Coleborne
School of Humanities and Social Science
University of Newcastle
Callaghan, NSW, Australia

Matthew Smith
Centre for the Social History of Health
and Healthcare
University of Strathclyde
Glasgow, UK

Covering all historical periods and geographical contexts, the series explores how mental illness has been understood, experienced, diagnosed, treated and contested. It will publish works that engage actively with contemporary debates related to mental health and, as such, will be of interest not only to historians, but also mental health professionals, patients and policy makers. With its focus on mental health, rather than just psychiatry, the series will endeavour to provide more patient-centred histories. Although this has long been an aim of health historians, it has not been realised, and this series aims to change that.

The scope of the series is kept as broad as possible to attract good quality proposals about all aspects of the history of mental health from all periods. The series emphasises interdisciplinary approaches to the field of study, and encourages short titles, longer works, collections, and titles which stretch the boundaries of academic publishing in new ways.

More information about this series at
http://www.palgrave.com/gp/series/14806

Sarah Ann Pinto

Lunatic Asylums in Colonial Bombay

Shackled Bodies, Unchained Minds

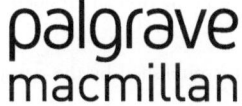

Sarah Ann Pinto
Independent Scholar
Wellington, New Zealand

Mental Health in Historical Perspective
ISBN 978-3-030-06818-9   ISBN 978-3-319-94244-5   (eBook)
https://doi.org/10.1007/978-3-319-94244-5

Cover illustration: Shackled Male Patient at Thana Lunatic Asylum, 1873-74, Author's illustration of a patient as described in the Annual Presidency Records (APR), 1873-74, p.4, National Library of Scotland

This Palgrave Macmillan imprint is published by the registered company Springer Nature Switzerland AG
The registered company address is: Gewerbestrasse 11, 6330 Cham, Switzerland

For
my parents
Susan Pinto and Julius Pinto
and
grandparents
Eva D'mello and Anthony D'mello
and
in
honour of
Mary

ACKNOWLEDGEMENTS

It takes a village to raise a child, or to write a book. I have had the support of a very multinational village while writing this book. From Professor Catherine Coleborne in Australia who encouraged me to publish my thesis, to relatives in London who opened their home to me, to my *whānau* in New Zealand and family in India—my village made this book possible. First, I thank Professor Catherine Coleborne for her feedback that has been crucial in editing this book. I thank my PhD supervisors, Professor Sekhar Bandyopadhyay and Dr. Giacomo Lichtner, for their constant support and guidance. Over the years, Dr. Fleur D'souza from my alma mater—St Xavier's College, Mumbai—has advised me in many ways. I thank her for recommending the topic, but most importantly for instilling in me a love for history and teaching.

The staff at the libraries, archives, and mental hospitals assisted me in many ways. These include the staff at the Victoria University of Wellington Library, Mumbai University Library, Heras Institute, Maharashtra State Archives, National Archives of India, British Library, Wellcome Institute, Ratnagiri Regional Mental Hospital, and the Thana Mental Hospital. At the Maharashtra State Archives, I thank Mrs. Swagata Salonke, Mr. D.D. Pawar, and Mrs. Joanna D'souza for the timely arrangement of the documents and assistant photographer Mr. Santosh Dhanawde for undertaking the mammoth task of digitizing the sources for me. I also thank Dr. Shubha Pandya for providing me copies of the *Bombay Gazette* and Mr. Shivade Nitin Mohan for helping me at the Thana Mental Hospital.

The archival and fieldwork was possible because of the hospitality of family and friends. In London, I thank my relatives Norma and Joe

D'mello for opening their home to me. I also thank Sr. Evelyn for providing me accommodation in Delhi. Despite my menial student budget, I could complete my archival and fieldwork because of their kindness.

This book has benefitted from various seminars and presentations. At the University of Mumbai, I thank Professors Manjari Kamat and Ruby Maloni for giving me the opportunity to present my research at the Department of History Research Symposium. I thank Professor Charlotte Macdonald for letting me present my research at the History Staff Seminar at the Victoria University of Wellington and Dr. Steve Behrendt for all the postgraduate seminars that helped me develop the skills I needed for the writing of this book.

The publishing team at Palgrave Macmillan's Mental Health in Historical Perspective Series were phenomenal. Molly Beck and Oliver Dyer made sure a young historian like me never felt like an orphan in the publishing world. The production team shared my vision for the book and swiftly designed and edited the manuscript like magic.

On a more personal note, I deeply value the support and prayers of my *whānau*. In Wellington, I thank the faculty and my fellow colleagues at the Victoria University's History Programme. Among my colleagues, Mark Dunick needs special mention for being my grammar guru. During the isolating writing phase, the friendship of Hannah, Chante, Angela, Damon, Eliza, Lucy, Severina and Maxy Vaz, Pexy and Manuel Miranda, Anastasia Rebello, and Fr. Vinay Kamath have been a great consolation. Since I began my research in 2014, Fr. Kevin O'Connors has been both a friend and a counsellor. Over cups of tea, he gave me both life lessons and research advice. I thank Raymond Pinto for mentoring me in matters of faith and social justice. I am also profoundly grateful to my dear friends Janice and Handricks Gayen for all the ways in which they have helped, that are too numerous to mention here.

Finally, I owe the deepest gratitude to my family. I am indebted to my grandparents Eva and Anthony D'mello for their endearing support. I thank my aunt and uncle, Jean and Prakash D'souza and cousin Sean for practically adopting me and for opening their home to me in New Zealand. To an amazing bunch of siblings who are my inspiration—Gerard, Rachel, Naomi, and Joel—thank you. To my parents, Julius and Susan Pinto, this book is the fruit of the numerous sacrifices you have made. Thanks Dad for travelling with me to the archives, libraries, hospitals, and Mum for being my personal manager in many ways. I thank you both for your unconditional love.

I dedicate this work to the people suffering from mental illness, their families, and those who work for their care.

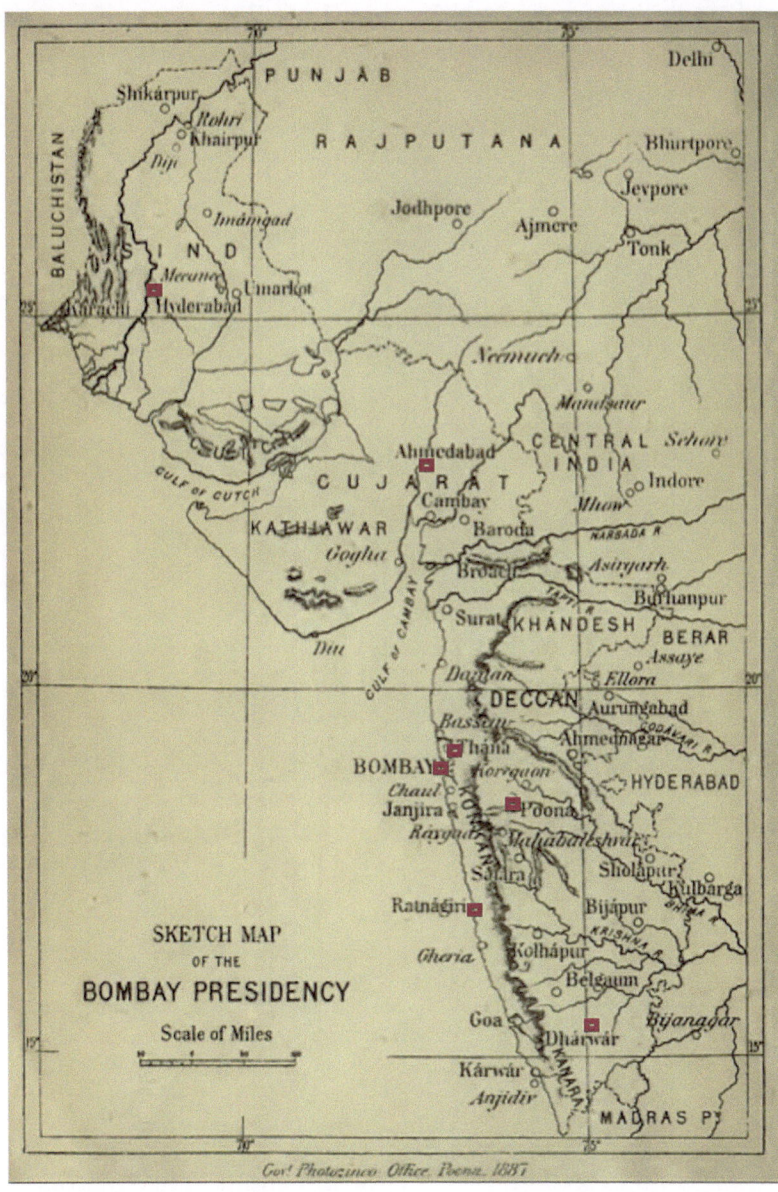

Lunatic Asylums in the Bombay Presidency, 1793–1921. (The map indicates the geographic locations only of the main asylums at Hyderabad, Ahmedabad, Thana, Colaba, Poona, Ratnagiri, and Dharwar [From North to South]. Source: Edmund Cox, *A Short History of the Bombay Presidency* (Bombay: Thacker and Co., 1887))

CONTENTS

ABBREVIATIONS

APR   Annual Administration and Progress Report
AR   Annual Report on the Mental Hospitals in the Bombay Presidency
Asst.   Assistant
BL   British Library
GD   General Department
GoB   Government of Bombay
GoI   Government of India
IMD   Indian Medical Department
IMS   Indian Medical Service
IOR   India Office Records
JD   Judicial Department
J–D   January to December
J–J   January to June
Lt. Col. Lieutenant Colonel
MSA   Maharashtra State Archives, Mumbai
NAI   National Archives of India, New Delhi
NLS   National Library of Scotland, Scotland
NMLA   Narotamdas Madhavdas Lunatic Asylum
Offg.   Officiating
PDD   Public Department Diary
PG   Pages
PWD   Public Works Department
RNP   Reports on Native Newspapers

LIST OF FIGURES

LIST OF TABLES

CHAPTER 1

Introduction

In the early hours of August 2001, the village of Erwadi in Tamil Nadu woke up to shrieks and wails. A freak fire had broken out at a shed on the precincts of the village shrine. The fire trapped 43 mentally ill people whom the shrine committee had chained there. Within minutes, the fire gutted the entire enclosure made of coconut palm branches. The fire killed 25 of the 43 people, including 11 women, that day.[1] After the accident, the government made an investigation into similar shrines that looked after mentally ill people in the State of Tamil Nadu. The government offered families that kept their relatives at such shrines places in mental hospitals. However, these families refused to have their relatives moved, choosing instead to keep them in 'sheds and chains'.[2] Even today, the shrine at Erwadi continues to house mentally ill people. A government-appointed psychiatrist has been visiting since May 2015, to provide medical intervention three times a week to those who were willing to avail of it. The medicines offered are a means to calm patients and to stop the shrine from using chains to restrain them.[3]

[1] *The Hindu*, 7 August 2001; http://www.thehindu.com/2001/08/07/stories/04072231.htm; accessed 21 October 2016.
[2] *The Hindu*, 26 August 2001; http:/www.thehindu.com/2001/08/26/stories/13260611.htm; accessed 21 October 2016.
[3] *The Hindu*, 16 May 2015; http:m.thehindu.com/news/national/tamilnadu/release-from-chains-at-erwadi-dargah-thanks-to-dawaduwa/article7213110.ece; accessed 21 October 2016.

© The Author(s) 2018
S. A. Pinto, *Lunatic Asylums in Colonial Bombay*,
Mental Health in Historical Perspective,
https://doi.org/10.1007/978-3-319-94244-5_1

The incident at Erwadi drew a considerable amount of public attention; the media labelled the local community as 'superstitious' because of its blind faith. The trend of labelling local communities as 'superstitious' is evident even in government mental health policies and programmes. Mental health programmes in India have primarily focused on offering 'scientific' methods of treatment to 'superstitious' families who refuse to have their relatives treated at hospitals and other health care centres.[4] The government and the media have conveniently blamed Indian society's superstitious beliefs for its poor response to mental hospitals; however, post-independence governments have paid little attention to providing effective mental health care to generate people's trust in it. In fact, India launched its first Mental Health Policy only in 2014.[5] Mental health care has remained peripheral to government health care policies and provisions.

The mental health care system and its clientele face several challenges in India. First, India's psychiatrist/patient ratio stands only at 0.3:100,000.[6] Second, government mental hospitals have frequently made headlines for the abuse of patients. The State of Maharashtra[7] has four government mental hospitals at Thana, Yerawada, Nagpur, and Ratnagiri. The paucity of psychiatrists has left these institutions chiefly under the management of untrained subordinate staff. The only educational qualification required of them is a primary education, and their posts are permanent.[8] In the hospitals at Thana and Yerawada, the media has reported several cases of abuse by subordinate staff. Patients sweep floors and even clean toilets, complying with orders from the staff to avoid abuse.[9] In 2007, a report by the Chief Judicial Magistrate exposed the poor conditions of the four hospitals regarding basic facilities like food, drainage, and water. The Indian

[4] *The Hindu*, 7 August 2001; http://www.thehindu.com/2001/08/07/stories/04072231.htm; accessed 21 October 2016.
[5] *Wall Street Journal*, 14 October 2014; http://blogs.wsj.com/indiarealtime/2014/10/14/indias-new-mental-health-policy-radical-but-tough-to-implement/; *Times of India*, 11 October 2014; http://timesofindia.indiatimes.com/india/Indias-first-mental-health-policy-launched/articleshow/44778494.cms; accessed 21 October 2016.
[6] *The Indian Express*, 20 May 2016; http://indianexpress.com/article/opinion/editorials/mental-illness-india-china-lancet-study-2809626/; accessed 21 October 2016.
[7] Most parts of Maharashtra came under the jurisdiction of the Bombay Presidency under colonial rule.
[8] *The Indian Express*, 23 December 2014; http://indianexpress.com/article/mumbai/in-urgent-need-of-being-human-mental-hospitals/; accessed 21 October 2016.
[9] Ibid.

government in the past has recognized the deplorable conditions within mental institutions. Recognizing that their nature was 'custodial', the government decided to bring them under 'comprehensive management'.[10]

Keeping in line with this vision, the government launched national and district mental health programmes in 1982. However, shortage of staff and resources greatly limited the success of the National Mental Health Programme (NMHP) and District Mental Health Programme (DMHP).[11] Shortage of resources and staff was only part of the problem. NMHP and DMHP aimed to 'modernise' psychiatric practices and create 'awareness' among Indian communities. Modernization implied implementation of western models of psychiatry, and 'awareness' meant making Indian communities accept 'modern' methods of treatment.[12]

Dr. Eduardo Duran, the Director of Health and Wellness for the United Auburn Indian Community in Northern California, has argued that such mental health policies and programmes that undermine indigenous spiritual beliefs, facilitate the continuation of 'neo-colonization' of indigenous peoples.[13] Exclusive western models have been largely unsuccessful in the mental healing process of American Indian communities. In fact, the continuance of such models has only served those in the existing system whose power positions it reinforces. Furthermore, these institutions become avenues for jobs only for those who agree with the continued colonization of indigenous peoples.[14] An examination of the history of these institutions brings to light continuing patterns of abuse within such institutions.

Psychiatric care in government mental institutions in India still bases itself on a colonial model. On my visit to the three hospitals in Maharashtra, the evidence clearly pointed to their custodial character. The colonial government constructed three of the four mental hospitals at Thana, Yerawada, and Ratnagiri. At Ratnagiri, a general physician from the government hospital oversaw the mental hospital. He held additional charge of the hospital,

[10] National Mental Health Programme, India, 1982; http://mohfw.nic.in/WriteRead Data/l892s/9903463892NMHP%20detail.pdf; accessed 21 October 2016.
[11] V. Sayee Kumar, 'School Mental Health Practice: Challenges for School Social Work in India', in Abraham P. Francis (ed.), *Social Work in Mental Health: Areas of Practice, Challenges, and Way Forward* (New Delhi, Singapore, London, California: Sage Publications, 2014), pp. 42–43.
[12] National Mental Health Program, India, 1982, pp. 1–2.
[13] Eduardo Duran, *Healing the Soul Wound: Counselling with American Indian and Other Native People* (New York: Teachers College Press, 2006), p. 14.
[14] Ibid., p. 25.

much like in the nineteenth century. The Ratnagiri Mental Hospital had no therapists. The former occupational therapy centre was now an empty locked room. At Ratnagiri and Yerawada, hospital staff employed patients in chores around the asylum. At the Thana Mental Hospital, one method of occupational therapy involved work on a weaving machine installed when the government inaugurated the asylum in 1902. Such conditions provide some obvious explanations why local communities avoid mental hospitals. The situation indicates that the Indian community's aversion to mental hospitals has some historical roots.

Dr. Duran, in his book *Healing the Soul Wounds*, postulated that colonial institutions left indigenous communities in America with historical traumas or 'soul wounds'. In the American Indian worldview, there is a holistic understanding of mental health: the mind, body, and spirit are interlinked. Therefore, colonial institutions, in the experiences of American Indians, affected their physical and psycho-spiritual wellbeing. Moreover, such trauma is intergenerational and has had an increasing negative implication for each subsequent generation.[15] Concerning colonial asylums in Bombay, such 'soul wounding' is evident in examples of the incarceration of Indians because of differences in colonial and Indian worldviews. In 1849, a magistrate in Ahmedabad sent Brahmin Devram to the asylum because he went on a religious fast. The magistrate concluded that the Brahmin's fast was an attempt at suicide and he admitted Devram to the Ahmedabad Asylum.[16] Such a misconstruction was just one example of a 'soul wound'. In addition, colonial asylums were in an appalling condition adding to the trauma of those who experienced life within them.

In 1904, Superintendent J.P. Barry described lunacy administration in India as the 'veritable Cinderella' in the family of colonial institutions.[17] He complained about meagre government funding for asylums. He also petitioned the government to stop the practice of charging fees for first-class paying patients, because: 'The entire building [was] more like a godown or a dilapidated barrack than an asylum. It [was] a shock to one's sense of justice to demand Rs. 4 a day for housing mentally sick people in

[15] Duran, *Healing the Soul Wound*, pp. 15–16.

[16] From the Magistrate of Ahmedabad to the Superintending Surgeon, Ahmedabad, 15 August 1849, Judicial Department (JD), Government of Bombay (GoB), General Department (GD), 1849/ 38, Maharashtra State Archives (MSA), Mumbai.

[17] From Lt. Col. J.P. Barry, Superintendent, Colaba Lunatic Asylum, to the Personal Asst. to the Surgeon General with the Government of Bombay, 25 June 1904, GoB, GD, 1907/81, MSA.

so unsuitable a place'.[18] While superintendents complained of lack of amenities and poor funding, they ironically criticized the reluctance of Indian communities to admit relatives to an asylum. Startling similarities are evident in situations regarding mental health treatment and Indian communities during colonial times and today, both in terms of government neglect and community aversion. There is therefore a need for a 'new narrative' of mental health treatment. Dr. Duran argued dealing with such historical issues was imperative to the writing of new narratives in mental health treatment.[19]

This book, then, is an attempt to deal with the historical issues associated with mental hospitals by bringing to light historical traumas or 'soul wounds' experienced by local communities as they encountered the colonial asylum system in the Bombay Presidency. The use of the term 'soul wound' is intentional. It does not imply a common conception of the 'soul' among communities in India. Rather, the study uses it to be inclusive of the 'sacred' beliefs integral to the understanding of the mind and mental health across various Indian communities.[20] In the experience of Indians, the lunatic asylum had implications on their physical, psychological, and spiritual wellbeing.

While violence and abuse within the asylum was a source of trauma to patients, the undermining of Indian worldviews, cultures, and beliefs further added to their wounding. 'Epistemic violence'[21] was common both within and outside the asylum, as local knowledge concerning mental health and treatment was designated as superstitious—as opposed to colonial knowledge that was deemed modern and scientific. These unresolved historical traumas are intergenerational.[22] Aversion to government mental hospitals or treatment programmes, this study argues, is not merely a result of superstition, but rather a consequence of historical traumas associated with the mental hospital. Dr. Duran has effectively treated his American Indian clientele by using this method, of first dealing with

---

[18] From Lt. Col. J.P. Barry, Superintendent, Colaba Lunatic Asylum, to the Personal Asst. to the Surgeon General with the Government of Bombay, 20 August 1904, GoB, GD, 1904/57, MSA.

[19] Duran, *Healing the Soul Wound*, p. 27.

[20] Sudhir Kakar, *Shamans, Mystics and Doctors* (Chicago: The University of Chicago Press, 1982), pp. 4–5.

[21] Gayatri Spivak, 'Can the Subaltern Speak?', in Cary Nelson and Lawrence Grossberg (eds.), *Marxism and the Interpretation of Culture* (London: Macmillan, 1988), p. 24.

[22] Duran, *Healing the Soul Wound*, p. 16.

historical issues and second, writing a new narrative in the field of mental health treatment which is inclusive of the indigenous worldview.[23] There is an urgent need for writing a 'new narrative' concerning mental health treatment in India. This book, in dealing with the historical issues, paves the way for that 'new narrative'.

The book addresses these historical issues by examining, as a case study, the colonial lunatic asylums in the Bombay Presidency. The Presidency presents an interesting case study for analysing the government's attitude towards lunacy administration. Of the three main presidencies—Bombay, Bengal, and Madras—the colonial government considered Bombay's lunatic asylums as least profitable to the state.[24] Moreover, superintendents in Bombay often accused the government of neglecting lunacy administration[25] Superintendents faced a huge challenge in managing such poorly funded asylums. However, Bombay's elite stepped in to fill the gap, donating huge amounts for the establishment of asylums.[26] Such public sponsorship from Bombay's elite towards lunatic asylums is peculiar to the Presidency. Yet, Bombay's elite, much like the other classes, did not use the asylum as a curative institution for their own relatives.

The government constantly highlighted the need 'to induce well-off natives to send their relatives to the asylum'.[27] However, the elite eluded the asylum because it lacked scientific methods of treatment. Besides, the poor segregation between 'criminal lunatics' and other patients at the Colaba Asylum was another factor that dissuaded them from the use of the asylum.[28] Asylum buildings were so poorly maintained that Superintendent J.P. Barry himself called the Colaba Asylum a 'godown or a dilapidated

---

[23] Duran, *Healing the Soul Wound*.

[24] From the Offg. Secretary to the Government of India to Secretary to the Government of Bombay, 13 August 1894, Government of India (GoI), Home Department, P 4554, India Office Records (IOR), British Library (BL), London.

[25] From Lt. Col. J.P. Barry, Superintendent, Colaba Lunatic Asylum to the Personal Asst. to the Surgeon General with the Government of Bombay, 25 June 1904, GoB, GD, 1907/81, MSA.

[26] Anil Kumar, *Medicine and the Raj: British Medical Policy in India, 1835–1911* (New Delhi: Altamira Press, 1998), p. 41.

[27] Annual Administration and Progress Report on the Lunatic Asylums in the Bombay Presidency (APR) for the Year 1874–1875, p. 15, National Library of Scotland (NLS), Scotland.

[28] Reports on Native Newspapers (RNP), *Jam-e-Jamshed*, 20 April 1889, K 416, January to December (J–D), pages (PG) 1–160, 1889, GoB, MSA. The *Jam-e-Jamshed* was a Gujarati weekly from Bombay.

barrack'.[29] The concerns of Bombay's elite were therefore not ill founded. The elite insisted that the government start 'private asylums'—'first class institution[s]' for 'well to do lunatics'.[30] The elite thus displayed a class bias in asylum matters through abstention from public asylums. The middle class and the poor also avoided the use of the asylum because of the stigma associated with the process of admission and incarceration. Most patients in the asylum were persons 'found committing mischief in the public streets and [were] caught and conveyed [to the asylum] by the police'.[31]

People across all classes in Bombay remained indifferent to the asylum system. As Superintendent J. Shaw explained, in India there was an 'absence of a definitely expressed public opinion' on asylum matters and a preference for 'indigenous systems'.[32] Because families preferred 'indigenous systems', they refused to admit relatives to an asylum despite having easy access to them. Bombay had an excellent transport system, especially in the second half of the nineteenth century. New railways connected the Presidency with its hinterlands.[33] Moreover, many of the asylums, especially in the nineteenth century, were centrally located. Yet, the asylum remained a place for the poor and destitute. Such asylum demographics were not a result of poor families willing to admit relatives. Even poor families refused to accept separation from mentally ill family members.[34]

Families, along with traditional practitioners and caretakers, took primary responsibility for the care of the mentally ill. Such traditional health practitioners and caretakers competed with the newly established asylum system. Bombay presents an interesting case study to analyse the dynamics between such traditional systems and the lunatic asylum. Asylum agencies particularly targeted traditional caretakers of the mentally ill like *fakirs*.[35]

[29] From Lt. Col. J.P. Barry, Superintendent, Colaba Lunatic Asylum to the Personal Asst. to the Surgeon General with the Government of Bombay, 20 August 1904, GoB, GD, 1904/57, MSA.

[30] RNP, *Jam-e-Jamshed*, 20 April 1889, K 416, J–D, PG 1–160, 1889, GoB, MSA. The *Jam-e-Jamshed* was a Gujarati weekly from Bombay.

[31] RNP, *Bombay Chabuk*, 13 July 1870, GD, K404/ 251, J–D, PG 1–543, GoB, MSA.

[32] W.S. Jagoe Shaw, 'The Alienist Department of India', *British Journal of Psychiatry*, Vol. 78, April 1932, p. 339.

[33] Ian J. Kerr, 'Representation and Representations of Railways of Colonial and Post-Colonial South Asia', *Modern Asian Studies*, Vol. 37, No. 2, 2003, p. 289.

[34] From the Civil Surgeon Dharwar to the Commissioner of Bombay, 3 August 1844, GoB, GD, 1844/34/380, MSA.

[35] A *Faqueer/Fakir* is an ascetic or a religious mendicant.

In Bombay's asylums, *fakirs* along with beggars and religious mendicants formed the largest patient population in lunatic asylums.[36] Even though the government discouraged the use of traditional methods, local communities preferred going to local doctors and healers. Several archival files contained government proceedings initiated by family members petitioning for either the release or transfer of their relatives.

Among colonial observers, Bombay was a socio-cultural middle ground.[37] Bombay, unlike the other presidencies of Madras and Bengal, had a common asylum at Colaba for Europeans and Indians for the whole of the nineteenth century.[38] All these positive factors had no significant impact on the response of Indian communities to the asylum. Bombay had all the necessary ingredients for colonial psychiatry and the asylum system to flourish. Yet, the asylum received a poor local response. Thus, the Bombay Presidency presents a unique case to explore the factors that caused the western asylum system to fail in a colonial context.

As a regional history of the asylum system in the Bombay Presidency, this book will be the first to construct a chronological history of lunatic asylums in that part of British India. It examines the history of asylums from 1793—when the government sanctioned the building of the first lunatic asylum in Bombay—up to 1921, after which the government changed the designation 'lunatic asylum' to 'mental hospital'.[39] In examining this period, the book argues that the asylum system failed to assimilate itself into Indian society and remained a failed colonial medical enterprise, despite the efforts of the government to propagate its use. Inmate numbers are a clear indication of both the failure of the system as well as Indian aversion towards the asylum. At the end of 1865, there were 353 inmates in the asylums of the Presidency. In 1880, the total asylum population stood at 646. However, in the closing years of the nineteenth century, asylum population rose only by about 10 per cent. By 1900, the

---

[36] The Annual Report in 1876 stated, 'Many fakirs and sepoys have been admitted'. APR, 1876, p. 26, NLS; Also see Table 2.1.

[37] Sir Wilson William Hunter, *Bombay 1885–1890: A Study in Indian Administration:* (London: H. Frowde; Bombay, B.M. Malabari, 1892), p. 14.

[38] Waltraud Ernst, 'Colonial Policies, Racial Politics and the Development of Psychiatric Institutions in the Early Nineteenth-Century British India', in Waltraud Ernst and Bernard Harris (eds.), *Race, Science and Medicine, 1700–1960* (London: Routledge, Taylor and Francis Group, 1999), pp. 88–89.

[39] W.S. Jagoe Shaw, 'The Alienist Department of India', *British Journal of Psychiatry*, Vol. 78, April 1932, p. 339.

number of inmates stood at just 759.[40] Most of these patients were 'wanderers with no friends'.[41] Families were rarely willing to admit relatives to the asylum, and it became an institution for the 'lowest of the low'.[42]

LITERATURE REVIEW

Over the centuries, a society's understanding of insanity has determined its response to people who were deemed mentally ill. This understanding, in turn, determined the management of mental illness and attitudes towards the mentally ill. The closing decades of the eighteenth century in Britain marked a significant development in society's perception of insanity and its response to the 'insane' persons. The establishment of asylums in Britain reflected the ideological change regarding mental illness in Victorian society. This change was rooted in the growing secularization of the seventeenth and eighteenth century. Victorian society, influenced by secular ideals, dissociated madness from original sin and perceived madness as treatable. The notion that madness was treatable eventually led to the starting of institutions for curing and managing madness. Eighteenth-century madhouses were precursors of Victorian asylums.[43]

The rise of the lunatic asylum in Victorian Britain aroused the curiosity of several historians and social scientists. Michel Foucault attributed the rise of asylums to society's need to organize madness and hide unreason.[44] He traced the development of institutional confinement to the seventeenth century when European societies incarcerated significant groups of the population whom they deemed as deviant[45]; he called this the 'great confinement'. Eventually, society segregated the mad from other deviants, leading to the creation of asylums. Asylums served to organize madness by reinforcing morality and 'ethical uniformity' on the patients.[46] Foucault

---

[40] James Mills, 'The History of Modern Psychiatry in India, 1858–1947', *History of Psychiatry*, Vol. 12, 2001, pp. 434–435.

[41] Report of the Indian Hemp Drugs Commission, 1894–1895, Vol. 1, p. 231, NLS.

[42] Asst. Surgeon Lunatic Asylum, Colaba, to the Secretary of the Medical Board, 21 February 1847, GoB, GD, 1847/41, MSA.

[43] Roy Porter, *Mind-Forg'd Menacles: A History of Madness in England from Restoration to the Regency* (London: Althone Press, 1987), pp. 277–279.

[44] Michel Foucault, *Madness and Civilization: A History of Insanity in the Age of Reason*, trans. Richard Howard (New York: Vintage Books, 2003).

[45] Foucault, *Madness and Civilization*, pp. 38–39.

[46] Ibid., pp. 251, 257.

postulated that the increasing use of asylums resulted from the spread of market principles, which deemed unproductive individuals dispensable. European asylums then functioned as a system of social control for such unproductive individuals.[47]

In a similar vein, Andrew Scull postulated that asylums served a disciplinary function. He argued that the segregation of those labelled as mentally ill in asylums was not a result of urbanization and industrialization. Instead, he argued that during the nineteenth century the influence of capitalist ideals led to the restructuring of societies and asylums were an outcome of that restructuring.[48] Asylums facilitated the internalization of self-discipline to create productive individuals within a society organized on such ideals.[49] Asylums also gave psychiatrists their legitimacy as professionals and experts of mental illness.[50] Several historians have, however, disagreed with Foucault and Scull's proposition that asylums merely functioned to discipline and control deviance.

Many scholars have instead proposed that the asylum had a curative purpose. Roy Porter argued that while treatment practices involved 'repressive control', experiences of patients varied according to their personal circumstances and class. Many of these 'strategies of control' played an important role in the emergence of modern psychiatry in England. For many, private asylums or madhouses provided medical care and an additional option for families to manage mental illness. He argued that asylums in England were ideally set up to help cure the mentally ill. He challenged the Foucauldian idea of the 'great confinement' in England in the eighteenth century.[51] Historian Petteri Pietikainen concurred with Porter on the idea of 'great confinement'. He also argued that asylums were well-intentioned for the treatment of the mentally ill. However, its advocates could not foresee the negative implications of such a system.[52]

---

[47] Michel Foucault, *History of Madness*, trans. Jonathan Murphy and Jean Khalifa (London: Routledge Taylor and Francis Group, 2006), p. 259; Foucault, *Madness and Civilization*, pp. 253–256.

[48] Andrew Scull, *Museums of Madness: The Social Organization of Insanity in Nineteenth-Century England* (London: Trinity Press, 1979), pp. 15, 48.

[49] Ibid., p. 113.

[50] Andrew Scull, 'From Madness to Mental Illness: Medical Men as Moral Entrepreneurs', *European Journal of Sociology*, Vol. 16, No. 2, 1975, p. 254.

[51] Porter, *Mind Forg'd*, pp. 277–281.

[52] Petteri Pietikainen, *Madness: A History* (London and New York: Routledge Taylor and Francis Group, 2015), pp. 89, 156.

William Parry-Jones and Leonard Smith's scholarship corresponds with the views of Porter and Pietikainen. Jones' research focused exclusively on private madhouses, which he argued were 'indispensable' to managing mental illness in the eighteenth and early nineteenth centuries. During this period, private madhouses made 'good provisions' especially for mentally ill persons from the upper and middle classes.[53] While Jones' work focused on private madhouses, Len Smith analysed public asylums. Smith contended that there was a growing awareness that 'madness' was not merely deviance; it constituted 'suffering' that affected persons experiencing it and their families. He added that the lunatic asylum was a form of treatment that combined 'care and custody' and the asylum was a place of constant 'tension' between the two principles.[54] The analysis of the nature of asylums as a curative or custodial institution has been an overarching theme in the historiography of asylums. As David Wright argued, most of the existing scholarship on British asylums centres on the history of psychiatry and therefore provides only a partial understanding of the character of the asylum.

Instead, he argued that an analysis of non-medical and government agencies was crucial to a better understanding of asylums. Wright has argued that families played a pivotal role in shaping the character of nineteenth-century asylums. He postulated that confinement was a long-term phenomenon related to changes in the rise of an industrial society and the paucity of informal caring networks. The use of the asylum was a 'strategic response of households to the stresses of industrialization'. The demand for asylum committals from families propelled the expansion of the asylum system in the nineteenth century.[55] Unlike the scholarship on British asylums, the historiography of colonial psychiatry in India fails to elaborate on the pivotal role of families in asylum confinement. Rather, the agency of family remains a parenthesis to the discussion of colonial knowledge and psychiatry. This book deviates from this historiographical trend by centring its discussion around the agency of the family and community.

---

[53] William Ll. Parry-Jones, *The Trade in Lunacy: A study of Private Madhouses in England in the Eighteenth and Nineteenth Centuries* (London: Routledge and Keenan Paul, 1972), pp. 283, 291.

[54] Leonard Smith, *Cure Comfort and Safe Custody* (London, New York: Leicester University Press, 1999), p. 5.

[55] David Wright, 'Getting Out of the Asylum: Understanding the Confinement of the Insane in the Nineteenth Century', *Social History of Medicine*, Vol. 10, No. 1, 1997, pp. 137, 143, 155.

Another major theme that scholars have focused on in their analysis of lunatic asylums is the implications of gender.

Historians have examined the extent to which asylum agencies feminized madness. Elaine Showalter contended that doctors in in England in the nineteenth and twentieth centuries predominantly perceived madness as a female condition.[56] Vieda Skultans, while agreeing with Showalter, presented evidence for the same from the writings of nineteenth-century psychiatrists and authors like Henry Maudsley and George Burrows.[57] However, Joan Busfield contradicted this argument. She argued that in the nineteenth century, a more detailed analysis of medical classification of mental illness emerged and it had gender assumptions, rather than an increasing feminization of madness.[58] The historiography of Victorian asylums encompasses several conventional and non-conventional themes. In comparison, the historiography of colonial psychiatry is a relatively new domain.

In the closing decades of the twentieth century, historians combined the trajectories of psychiatry and colonialism, analysing the role of psychiatry in the Empire. In the years that followed, in the context of the British Empire, a growing scholarship emerged on colonial asylums in Africa, the British Caribbean, Fiji, Australia, New Zealand, Ireland, Canada, and India. Colonial psychiatry in Africa received its fair share of attention from historians like Jock McCulloh, Jonathan Sadowsky, Sally Swartz, Megan Vaughan, Julie Parle, and Harriet Deacon.[59]

Colonial ideation of race and mental illness is a dominant theme in the historiography of colonial psychiatry in Africa. Colonial theories presented

[56] Showalter, *Female Malady.*

[57] Vieda Skultans, *Madness and Morals: Ideas on Insanity in the Nineteenth Century* (London: Routledge and Kegan Paul, 1975), pp. 223–240.

[58] Joan Busfield, 'The Female Malady? Men, Women and Madness in Nineteenth-Century Britain', *Sociology*, Vol. 28, No. 1, 1994, p. 276.

[59] Jock McCulloh, *Colonial Psychiatry and The African Mind* (Cambridge: University Press, 1995); Jonathan Sadowsky, *Imperial Bedlam: Institutions of Madness in Colonial Southwest Nigeria* (Berkeley: University of California Press, 1999); Sally Swartz, 'The Black Insane in Cape, 1891–1920', *Journal of Southern African Studies*, Vol. 21, No. 3, September 1995, pp. 399–415; Megan Vaughan, *Curing their Ills: Colonial Power and African Illness* (California: Stanford University Press, 1991); Julie Parle, 'Witchcraft or Madness? The Amandiki of Zululand, 1894–1914', *Journal of Southern African Studies*, Vol 29, No. 1, March 2003, pp. 105–132; Harriet Deacon, 'Insanity, Institutions and Society: the Case of the Robben Island Lunatic Asylum, 1846–1910', in Roy Porter and David Wright (eds.), *The Confinement of the Insane: International Perspectives, 1800–1965* (New York: Cambridge University Press, 2003), pp. 20–53.

race as intrinsically connected to madness, and they used indigenous madness to back the theory of the white man's burden to civilize the African colony. Jock McCulloh argued that European colonies were the spawning grounds for the new science of ethnopsychiatry and eventually it worked to legitimize colonialism because it considered Africans incapable of governing themselves. He proposed that the most enduring legacy of ethnopsychiatry was the creation of 'the figure of a colonial subject'. McCulloh further added that the ethnopsychiatrist who belonged to the 'declining colonial class' used the knowledge of psychiatry, medicine, and the production of knowledge to keep the Africans subjugated.[60]

Even in the colonies, colonial authorities used psychiatry as a means of social control. Jonathan Sadowsky examined the colonial asylums in Nigeria and argued that status and cultural differences determined the extent of control exerted on indigenous patients.[61] Furthermore, he added that colonial psychiatric theory in Nigeria was more 'liberal' compared to other African colonies despite its racial overtones.[62] He also contended that though the government established lunatic asylums in Nigeria in 1906, for the first few decades the government was negligent and did not invest in improving treatment. Sadowsky claimed that the condition of Nigerian asylums were so bad that they were 'functionally equivalent' to prisons. Treatment methods and asylum conditions only improved post-independence because of the initiatives of Nigerian doctors.[63] Like Sadowsky, Swartz used the sociological category of race to analyse its implications on the treatment of patients in South Africa.

Swartz argued that racial classification was a critical in the management of asylums in the Cape Colony from its inception in 1846.[64] By the twentieth century, many fully segregated asylums were established. Colonial discourses produced during this period justified this segregation. Within the asylum, authorities 'stripped' black patients of their identities by labelling them with aetiological constructions of mental illness that were not part of African culture. Concerning asylum population, 'natives' formed a

[60] McCulloh, *Colonial Psychiatry and the African Mind*, pp. 1, 146, 144.

[61] Sadowsky, *Imperial Bedlam*, p. 5.

[62] Jonathan Sadowsky, 'Psychiatry and Colonial Ideology in Nigeria', *Bulletin of the History of Medicine*, Vol. 71, No. 1, 1997, p. 95.

[63] Ibid; Jonathan Sadowsky, 'Confinement and Colonialism in Nigeria', in Roy Porter and David Wright (eds.), *The Confinement of the Insane: International Perspectives, 1800–1965* (New York: Cambridge University Press, 2003), pp. 302, 309, 310.

[64] Swartz, 'The Black Insane in Cape', pp. 399–400, 402.

smaller number compared to whites. Colonial authorities explained this disparity as resulting from the primitive nature of 'natives', which made them less susceptible to mental illness.[65] In terms of classification of patients, along with race, gender played an important role. Asylum authorities enforced gendered segregation by maintaining separate wards and ensuring strict surveillance of patient social interactions.[66] In terms of diagnosis and treatment, Swartz argued that doctors were prejudiced in their understanding of black patients' illnesses. They made several presumptions about black persons and their illness. Moreover, racial biases even obscured their understanding of distinction between black 'sane' and 'insane'. Colonial psychiatry thus played a crucial role in legitimizing colonial rule by constructing the African as 'primitive, unrestrained physically, childish, hypersexual and potentially violent'.[67] Historian Megan Vaughan has also analysed the impact of such colonial constructions of a black identity and the production of colonial knowledge within colonial medical institutions. Vaughan examined colonial processes through which colonial agencies constructed meanings of insanity in an African colony. Tracing the growth of biomedicine and its use in the construction of an African identity in Nyasaland, she postulated that the construction of the identity of the African as different from that of the European served colonial purposes. Even colonial psychiatry maintained this idea of difference by engaging in 'pathologizing the "normal" African'. Such pathologizing categorized the mad African man or woman based on their non-conformity to the colonial construction of African identity. Asylum doctors considered African non-conformity as 'deculturation', since it erased existing boundaries of difference between the African and the European. The discourse on differences kept changing over time, leading to a change in concepts of normality and insanity of Africans. Additionally, Vaughan argued that even though a more elaborate classification of mental illness emerged in the twentieth century, treatment practices remained unchanged. Based on the number of Africans admitted, she disagreed with the Foucauldian proposition of the 'great confinement'. Yet, she contended that African lunatic asylums, largely because of the shortage of funds, remained mere places of confinement.[68]

---

[65] Swartz, 'The Black Insane in Cape', p. 409.

[66] Sally Swartz, 'Lost Lives: Gender, History and Mental Illness in the Cape', *Feminism and Psychology*, Vol. 9, No. 2, 1999, p. 154.

[67] Swartz, 'Black Insane in Cape', p. 415.

[68] Vaughan, *Curing their Ills*, pp. 12, 13, 118, 120.

Harriet Deacon, in her research on the Robben Island Lunatic Asylum in Cape Colony, made a similar argument about the custodial character of lunatic asylums. She contended that colonists perceived black insanity as disruptive to colonial order. However, indigenous mentally ill who lived in separate communities, geographically distant from white communities, were of little concern to colonial authorities. There was therefore no 'great confinement'. Patients who found themselves admitted were usually single black males who were criminal lunatics or had no community assistance. In the Cape Colony, many communities like the Africans, Khoisan, and Muslims preferred to use indigenous healing methods and avoided the use of the asylum. Even among the poor, the community's perceptions affected their use of the asylum. Moreover, the rigidity of asylum practices and a lack of accommodation of the cultural practices of non-Christian communities kept locals from using the asylum.[69] Likewise, Julie Parle in her research on asylums in Zululand argued that for locals, colonial psychiatry and western treatment methods were the last port of call for treating mentally ill relatives.[70] These findings are also applicable in the Indian context since in India cultural perceptions of the asylum affected the use of the asylum. Moreover, families who used the asylum did so as a last resort. This study highlights the role of community attitudes and perceptions of the asylum in shaping a family's willingness to admit relatives.

The central focus of scholarship on colonial psychiatry in Africa is the use of race in the categorization of mental illness among indigenous people and the use of western science and medicine in exerting control over African colonies. However, the scholarship on the relationship between colonial psychiatry and indigenous treatment methods is sparse, and there is a lacuna in present scholarship in exploring themes like asylum soundscapes and architecture. While historians have been adding to the historiography of African asylums over the last few decades, they have examined the history of lunatic asylums in the British Caribbean only recently.

Historian Leonard Smith argued that while the government intended Caribbean lunatic asylums for both treatment of patients and public safety, they largely performed a custodial function. By the mid-nineteenth century, these asylums were in a deplorable condition. Smith added that these poorly maintained asylums reflected the attitudes of an elite society

---

[69] Deacon, 'Insanity, Institutions and Society', pp. 52–53.

[70] Julie Parle, 'States of Mind: Mental illness and the quest for mental health in Natal and Zululand, 1868–1918', PhD Thesis, University of KwaZulu-Natal, 2004, p. viii.

towards black and coloured peoples, especially 'criminals, coolies and a low type of insane poor'. In these asylums doctors insisted on classification among white and black and coloured patients, since doctors perceived coloured and black patients as people with 'ingovernable passions' who were 'savage' in their habits. They therefore advocated moral management as a method of treatment to 'civilise' the 'native'. Despite advocating moral management, the government managed these asylums ineffectively. The Kingston Asylum in Jamaica became a public scandal in the 1860s. Subordinate staff who were untrained largely managed these asylums. In many instances, former patients served as staff.[71] An examination of the agency of asylum staff reveals a 'dismal tale of corruption and cruelty'. Moreover, these asylums were unhygienic, poorly equipped, and improperly maintained.[72] After the scandal became public, the government made a few improvements. Nevertheless, poor funding and overcrowding caused these improvements to last only temporarily. Provisions for patients remained at the most 'basic level'.[73] The scandal led to an increase in systematic regulation of asylums across the British Empire.[74] However, such regulations that led to improvements are not evident in Indian asylums. The scholarship on asylums in the British Caribbean has several gaps, including the implications of gender in treatment, indigenous treatment methods, and its relation to the colonial system and the agency of families. The meagre scholarship on asylums in the British Caribbean contrasts with the vast scholarship available on asylums in the Pacific colonies. This scholarship has adhered to the notion that the asylum was a means to discipline, but it deviated from the Foucauldian idea of 'great confinement'.

Historian Jaqueline Leckie researched asylums in colonial Fiji. She argued that there was no 'great confinement' in Fiji. Leckie's analysis of the Fijian asylum depicts it as a gendered space that served as a means of social control. She argued that Fijians used colonial asylums to discipline anyone who violated 'customary codes'. She attributed this acceptance of

---

[71] Leonard Smith, *Insanity, Race and Colonialism: Managing Mental Disorder in the Post-Emancipation British Caribbean, 1838–1914* (London: Palgrave Macmillan, 2014), pp. 30, 153–154, 173, 192.

[72] Sally Swartz, 'The Regulation of British Colonial Lunatic Asylums and the Origins of Colonial Psychiatry, 1860–1864', *American Psychological Association*, Vol. 13, No. 2, 2010, p. 167.

[73] Smith, *Insanity, Race and Colonalism*, pp. 75, 97.

[74] Swartz, 'The Regulation of British Colonial Lunatic Asylums', p. 160.

the asylum to an acceptance of colonial construction of indigenous madness. By the early twentieth century, families increasingly admitted their mentally ill relatives to the asylum.[75] In the Fijian context, the adoption of Christianity by Fijian families also affected their willingness to admit relatives. Families played an important role in the committal process.[76]

Catharine Coleborne's work on asylums in Australasia pays particular attention to the agency of families in the admission process. Coleborne analysed the role of asylums in settler colonies of Australia and New Zealand, where asylums served a communal function. She argued that families in Australia relied on the asylum for the care of their relatives who suffered from mental illness and even used it to mediate family conflicts.[77] The asylum system, in her view, worked in conjunction with the penal department as a means of social control. Stephen Garton's research on asylums in New South Wales also highlights the role of asylums in social policing. Women, in particular, became 'prime targets' of this policing. While the asylum was a system of control, in his view, it also served as a 'welcome break' for individuals who came from dysfunctional families. A major drawback if Garton's work is the absence of a narrative of the experiences of indigenous patients and families.[78] Coleborne's research has filled this lacuna to some extent. In her book *Madness in the Family*, she highlighted the victimization of Maori in New Zealand by colonial agencies and the undermining of traditional doctors by the colonial asylum system.[79]

While Coleborne's research focused on the interaction between families, communities, and the asylums, Dolly Mackinnon analysed asylum soundscapes in Australia. She used the aural environment of the asylums as evidence of the function of the asylum as a disciplinary institution.[80]

---

[75] Jacqueline Leckie, 'Modernity and Management of Madness in Colonial Fiji', *Paideuma*, Vol. 50, 2004, pp. 260–261, 263, 267–268.

[76] Weir discusses the spread of Christianity in Fiji. See Christine Weir, '"We Visit the Colo Towns … when it is Safe to Go": Indigenous Adoption of Methodist Christianity in the Wainibuka and Wainimala Valleys, Fiji, in the 1870s', *The Journal of Pacific History*, Vol. 49, No.2, 2014, pp. 129–150.

[77] Catharine Coleborne, *Madness in the Family: Insanity and Institutions in the Australasian Colonial World, 1860–1914* (UK: Palgrave Macmillan, 2010), p. 120.

[78] Stephen Garton, *Medicine and Madness: a Social History of Insanity in New South Wales, 1880–1940* (Kensington: New South Wales University Press, 1988), pp. 188–189.

[79] Coleborne, *Madness in the Family*, p. 62.

[80] Dolly Mackinnon, 'Hearing Madness the Soundscape of the Asylum', in Catharine Coleborne and Dolly Mackinnon (eds.), *Madness in Australia: Histories, Heritage and the Asylum* (Queensland: University of Queensland Press, 2003), pp. 73–82.

Additionally, she analysed the therapeutic role of music in Australian asylums. MacKinnon was the first to initiate a discussion on asylum soundscapes.[81] However, she generalized that asylum soundscapes were 'regulated and regimented' in all British colonial asylums around the world.[82] As argued in this book, such a theory is irrelevant to asylums in colonial India. The historiography of asylums in Australia and New Zealand largely focuses on the asylum as an institution of social control and discipline, and the agency of families in the committal process. The acceptance of families of the asylum as a medical institution directly influenced admission numbers. The historiography of Irish asylum presents a similar narrative on the role of families.

In Ireland, Mark Finnane argued, asylums were a source of relief for families. They became an 'indispensable part' of the social order. Administrative and judicial authorities committed patients to an asylum based on several factors. The variations in the causes of admission displayed the lack of clarity among asylum agencies regarding the purpose of the asylum. Irish families did not challenge these committals since they trusted the efficacy of the asylum. While asylums initially housed the poor, by the end of the nineteenth century, doctors treated patients from all classes.[83] According to Elizabeth Malcolm, families willingly negotiated committal of relatives with asylum agencies, eventually causing the overcrowding of Irish asylums.[84] Irish families perceived the asylum as benefiting the safety of the family and neighbourhood.[85] This perception or 'popular mentality' played an important role in the 'image and use' of the asylum.[86] Families and the government (quasi-colonial government) intended the asylum as a humanitarian effort to help the mentally ill. However, a lack of professionalization, overcrowding and 'brutality' of

---

[81] Dolly Mackinnon, "'Jolly and Fond of Singing": The Gendered Nature of Musical Entertainment in Queensland Mental Institutions, c1870–1937', in Coleborne and Mackinnon (eds.), *Madness in Australia*, pp. 157–168.

[82] Mackinnon, 'Hearing Madness', p. 75.

[83] Mark Finnane, *Insanity and the Insane in Post-Famine Ireland* (New Jersey: Barnes and Noble, 1981), pp. 13, 15–16, 223.

[84] Elizabeth Malcolm, "'Ireland's crowded Madhouses": the Institutional Confinement of the Insane in Nineteenth- and Twentieth-Century Ireland', in Roy Porter and David-Wright (eds.), *The Confinement of the Insane: International Perspectives, 1800–1965* (New York: Cambridge University Press, 2003), p. 333.

[85] Finnane, *Insanity and the Insane*, p. 15.

[86] Mark Finnane, 'Asylums, Families and the State', *History Workshop Journal*, No. 20, Autumn, 1985, p. 145.

asylum agencies greatly limited these humanitarian concerns. This study similarly focuses on the agency of Indian families in the process of admission and release of patients in the Indian context. It also analyses the extent to which 'popular mentality' affected the use of the asylum.

In British Canada, 'popular mentality' also affected the community's use of the asylum. Initially, Canadian families used the asylum as a last resort because of the stigma associated with it.[87] However, by the late nineteenth century these families began to perceive the asylum as a curative institution. This perception facilitated their increasing use of the asylum. In Canada, committal happened through two processes. The first was the civil stream, which required the family to get the signatures of three doctors and the mayor. The second route to asylum committal was an order from a justice of peace. Families used the civil stream to 'negotiate' with asylum doctors about the admission process.[88] Patients admitted by families came from varying ethnic, geographic, and socio-economic backgrounds.[89] Canadian asylums, like Irish and Australasian asylums, became the 'arbiter of social and familial conflict'.[90] This book explores the reasons for the failure of the Indian asylum system in mediating social and familial conflict. Instead, as this study postulates, the asylum added to the trauma experienced by families. The themes discussed by scholars on psychiatry in Britain and her colonies have been examined by historians of colonial psychiatry in India.

Shridhar Sharma and L.P. Varma have provided a brief descriptive history of mental hospitals in India from 1784 to 1947.[91] They divided the development of mental hospitals into four phases: the initial phase from 1784 to 1857; the second phase from 1858 to the early nineteenth

---

[87] James Moran, *Committed to the State Asylum: Insanity and Society in Nineteenth-Century Quebec and Ontario* (Montreal & Kingston, London, Ithaca: McGill-Queen's University Press, 2001), pp. 78, 97–98, 115.

[88] Bartlett argued that unlike in England, the absence of a poor law in Canada facilitated the direct admission of patients by families. See Peter Bartlett, 'Structures of Confinement in nineteenth-Century Asylums', *International Journal of Law and Psychiatry*, Vol. 23, No. 1, 2000, pp. 10–11.

[89] David Wright, Laurie Jacklin, Tom Themeles, 'Dying to Get Out of the Asylum: Mortality and Madness in Four Mental Hospitals in Victorian Canada, c. 1841–1891', *Bulletin of the History of Medicine*, Vol. 87, No. 4, 2013, p. 618.

[90] Moran, *Committed to the Asylum*, p. 115; Finnane, 'Asylums, Family and the State', p. 143; Coleman, *Madness in the Family*, p. 120.

[91] Shridhar Sharma and L.P. Varma, 'History of Mental Hospitals in the Indian Subcontinent', *Indian Journal of Psychiatry*, Vol. 26, No. 4, pp. 295–300.

century; the third phase, which was categorized from the early nineteenth century to 1920; and the final phase from 1920 until 1947. Their work mainly provides a chronological timeline of establishment and expansion of mental hospitals in India. As for the nature of colonial asylums, Sharma concluded that asylums were mere 'detention' sites.[92]

Waltraud Ernst has also made a similar proposition; in her opinion, colonial asylums were 'temporary receptacles' that were eventually trans-formed into 'total institutions'.[93] She postulated that the Raj used colonial psychiatry to legitimize its 'socio-political infrastructure' and served to validate its humanitarian role in India. Through the maintenance of these mental institutions and the introduction of western psychiatry, the colo-nists could persuade the colonized into believing in the myth of British supremacy and the need for the colonized to continue their dependence on the Raj.[94] She argued that the categories of race and class shaped the internal organization of Bombay's asylums.[95] Ernst's work features the most extensive scholarship on colonial Indian asylums; however, her writ-ings mostly focus on European patients. Moreover, she rarely engages with the themes of the categorization and treatment of patients in *mofus-sil*[96] asylums in the Bombay Presidency. Her study of asylums in Bombay does not use sources from the Maharashtra State Archives (MSA). Apart from Ernst' historical work, historian James Mills has authored several works on colonial asylums in India. Mills, however, contradicts Ernst's conclusion that colonial asylums were 'temporary receptacles'.

Instead, Mills has proposed that Indian asylums provided modern methods of treatment.[97] The purpose of treatment regimes was to civilize Indians rather than colonize them.[98] The civilizing process functioned to

---

[92] Shridhar Sharma, *Mental Hospitals in India* (New Delhi: Director General of Health Services, 1990), p. 52.

[93] Waltraud Ernst, *Mad Tales from the Raj: Colonial Psychiatry in South Asia, 1800–58* (New York: Anthem Press, 2010), p. 126.

[94] Ibid., p. xv.

[95] Waltraud Ernst, 'Racial, Social and Cultural Factors in the Development of a Colonial Institution: The Bombay Lunatic Asylum (1670–1858)', *Internationales Asienforum*, Vol. 22, No. 3–4, 1991, pp. 61–80.

[96] Areas outside the main urban centers of the Presidency.

[97] James Mills, *Madness, Cannabis and Colonialism: The 'Native-Only' Lunatic Asylums of British India, 1857–1900* (Basingstoke: Macmillan Press Limited, 2000), pp. 103–104.

[98] James Mills, '"More Important to Civilise than Subdue"? Lunatic Asylums, Psychiatric Practice and Fantasies of the "Civilising Mission" in British India 1858—1900', in Harald Fischer-Tiné and Michael Mann (eds.), *Colonialism as Civilising Mission* (London: Anthem Press, 2003), pp. 171–190.

produce bodies that could prove useful to the colonial system.[99] He analysed the nature of asylums in the latter half of the nineteenth century and contended that 'native' asylums became sites of colonial knowledge production. Knowledge produced from these asylums served as common knowledge about Indian people. In elaborating the argument, he used the example of patients who were hemp users. After observing these patients, doctors drew conclusions on the use of hemp and its effects. Hemp users in asylums became representatives of hemp users in India. Colonial authorities linked hemp to insanity and insanity to violence. Such knowledge produced in colonial asylums about insanity, hemp, and its links to violence served as infallible truths for colonial officers.[100] Mills' writing also highlights Indian responses to the asylum. He argued that local families used the asylum to discipline family members.[101] He added that Indian families only temporarily 'banished' their relatives to an asylum; families took back their relatives since they had productive value.[102] His conclusion evaluates Indian responses based on a western capitalist ideal of productivity. This book instead argues that the community-centric nature of Indian society made the asylum an alien institution. Disagreeing with Mills' proposition that asylums were not merely 'detention sites',[103] the book contends that asylums in Bombay were places of confinement that largely lacked provisions of modern psychiatric treatment. Colonial doctors themselves called asylums mere 'lock-ups'.[104] Mills' writing also contains a few geographic inaccuracies. He places the asylums at Ahmedabad and Colaba in the Bengal Presidency,[105] while these areas were parts of the Bombay Presidency.

Adding to the extensive scholarship of Ernst and Mills are the works of Shruti Kapila, Shilpi Rajpal, and Anouska Bhattacharyya. Kapila uses the case study of Bombay to write a 'biography of colonial psychiatry'. She argued that colonial psychiatry was linked to colonial governmentality and it was informed by the dual motivations of maintaining order and a

---

[99] Mills, *Madness, Cannabis and Colonialism*, p. 112.

[100] Ibid., pp. 36, 53.

[101] James Mills, 'Psychiatry on Edge? Vagrants, Families, and Colonial Asylums in India, 1857–1900', in Sameetah Agha and Elizabeth Kolsky (eds.), *Fringes of Empire* (New Delhi, Oxford University Press, 2009), p. 201.

[102] Mills, *Madness, Cannabis and Colonialism*, p. 140.

[103] Ibid., pp. 103–104.

[104] From the Surgeon General with the Government of Bombay to the Secretary to the Government, Government of Bombay, 5 November 1904, GoB, GD, 1905/55, MSA.

[105] Mills, *Madness, Cannabis and Colonialism*, p. 186.

humanitarian concern. She attributed the expansion of the asylum system in the second half of the century to the 'processes of urbanization' and the 'colonial management of public spaces'. Colonial psychiatry, she argued, failed to evolve into a specialized profession because of the imperatives of colonial governmentality and financial expediency. Civilization was the main sociological category used by colonial psychiatrists.[106] Kapila's research presents intriguing evidence of the links between governmentality and colonial psychiatry. However, the exclusive focus on colonial psychiatry excludes the everyday workings of the asylum. Moreover, while the superintendent receives a fair share of attention for his agency, she fails to discuss the role of other agencies, especially Indian staff in the development of colonial psychiatry. The chronological framework does not permit a comparison with asylums that existed prior to 1849, and this prevents a proper analysis of what seems like an intentional 'proliferation' of asylums in Bombay. First, asylums built at Poona and Ahmedabad were only replacements for the older asylums that existed prior to this period. Additionally, public donations funded the building of the other asylums, with the exception of the Ratnagiri Lunatic Asylum. The government's lunacy policy was 'intentional', but that 'intentionality' lacked the zeal that clearly characterized western medicine and public health.[107] This book therefore, in analysing Bombay's asylum system from 1793 to 1921, provides a macro perspective to the establishment and expansion of the asylum system in Bombay. While colonial psychiatry effectively employed 'civilization' as a sociological category, a closer analysis of Annual Reports demonstrates that race was equally important. Colonial agencies, as this study argues, used race to justify differential treatment of Indian and European patients. Overall, Kapila's research tactfully tackles the questions surrounding the development of colonial psychiatry.

Shilpi Rajpal and Anouska Bhattacharyya have also shared Kapila's focus on colonial psychiatry. Their works focused on the James Clark Enquiry of 1868—an initiative by the Government of India to make a comprehensive study of the condition of lunatic asylums in India. However, the enquiry only covered 14 asylums in India; it completely excluded Bombay's lunatic

---

[106] Shruti Kapila, 'The Making of Colonial Psychiatry, Bombay Presidency, 1849–1940', Ph.D Thesis, School of Oriental and African Studies, University of London, 2002, pp. 28, 30–31, 263.

[107] David Arnold, 'Public Health and Public Power: Medicine and Hegemony in Colonial India', in Daglar Engles and Shula Marks (eds.), *Contesting Colonial Hegemony: State and Society in Africa and India* (London, New York: British Academic Press, 1994), p. 142.

asylums. The main source of the enquiry was a questionnaire for superintendents regarding the lunatic asylums under their charge. Rajpal argued that though the enquiry reflected a humanitarian concern, it did not bring about any radical reform to lunacy administration in India.[108] On the nature of asylums, Rajpal postulated that they were punitive and regulatory institutions.[109] Bhattacharyya also evaluated the James Clark Enquiry and contended that it was a means to gain information on the 'superintendent's everyday life'.[110] On the nature of 'native' lunatic asylums, she postulated that they were 'permeable' spaces with hybrid treatment practices. The government permitted 'oligopoly' in 'native' lunatic asylums because it lacked medical expertise.[111] However, by the twentieth century, these asylums transformed into 'bastions of colonial hegemony'.[112] The hybrid asylum environment changed into a homogenized colonial medical institution. This transformation, she argued, was a result of the professionalization of western psychiatry in Europe and lunacy legislation. For example, the Lunacy Act of 1912 paved the way for a change in the designation of lunatic asylum to mental hospital.[113] Bhattacharyya, however, fails to consider that the change in designation of lunatic asylums to 'mental hospitals' was met with strong opposition from superintendents across India.[114] Bhattacharyya also ignores the local or regional variations of the asylums in India. The degree of transformation of the asylums into a 'colonial archetype' depended on such variables as the superintendents, availability of funds, and support of the presidency governments. Moreover, it analyses themes like the asylum soundscape and use of clothing as treatment that are missing from the extant scholarship on India.

Another important theme explored to some extent by scholars is the dynamics between traditional healing systems and western psychiatry and

[108] Shilpi Rajpal, 'Colonial Psychiatry in Mid-Nineteenth Century India: The James Clark Enquiry', *South Asia Research*, Vol. 35, No. 1, 2015, p. 76.
[109] Rajpal, 'Colonial Psychiatry', pp. 61–80; Shilpi Rajpal, 'Quotidian Madness: Time, Management and Asylums in Colonial North India', *Studies in History*, Vol. 31, No 2, p. 221.
[110] Anouska Bhattacharyya, 'Indian Insanes, Lunacy in the "Native" Asylums of Colonial India, 1858–1912', PhD Thesis, Harvard University, 2013, p. 142.
[111] Ibid., p. 131.
[112] Ibid., p. 211.
[113] Bhattacharyya, 'Indian Insanes, Lunacy in the "Native" Asylums of Colonial India', p. 188.
[114] From the Superintendent, Central Lunatic Asylum Yerawada, to the Surgeon General with the Government of Bombay, GoB, GD, 1922/2257-B, MSA.

the asylum system. Mitchell Weiss has argued that cohabitation, some interaction, and an intense competition characterized the relationship between the two systems.[115] Likewise, Sanjeev Jain contended that until the early nineteenth century there was an exchange of ideas, medicines, and techniques between healing traditions of India and Britain. However, scientific advances caused the two to become distant.[116] Sudhir Kakar also researched the relationship between western and traditional healing methods. He provides an interesting analysis in his book *Shamans, Mystics and Doctors* about the relation between western psychiatry and healing practices in contemporary India. He argued that there were several resemblances between western psychoanalysis and traditional mental health treatment methods in India. He added that the greatest difference between the two was that unlike psychoanalysis that excluded the 'sacred', the 'sacred' was an integral part of healing treatment in Indian healing systems.[117] While Kakar's work provides a deep understanding of Indian healing traditions, his work is a psychoanalytical analysis rather than a historical one. There is a lacuna in the scholarship concerning the relationship between asylums and Indian mental health systems during the colonial period.

The historiography of colonial psychiatry primarily veers towards an analysis of colonial motivation for starting asylums, its use as a means of social control, and legitimization of colonial rule. Historians of colonial medicine have adopted a similar approach. Colonial medical historians have intensely engaged in a debate over the motivations behind the establishment of colonial medical institutions. Some historians adhere to the notion that colonial medicine was a 'tool of the Empire' since it served to legitimize colonialism. The state also used it as a means to penetrate deeper into Indian social life.[118] Deviating from this view, David Arnold argued that western medicine served a far more complex function, serving both

---

[115] Mitchell Weiss, 'The Treatment of Insane Patients in India in the Lunatic Asylums of the Nineteenth Century', *Indian Journal of Psychiatry*, Vol. 25, No. 4, 1983, p. 315.

[116] Sanjeev Jain, 'Psychiatry and Confinement in India', in Roy Porter and David Wright (eds.), *The Confinement of the Insane: International Perspectives, 1800–1965* (New York: Cambridge University Press, 2003), p. 296.

[117] Kakar, *Shamans, Mystics and Doctors*, pp. 1–4.

[118] Satadru Sen, 'The Savage Family: Colonialism and Female Infanticide in Nineteenth-Century India', *Journal of Women's History*, Vol. 14, No. 3, Autumn 2002, p. 75; Daniel R. Headrick, *The Tools of Empire: Technology and European Imperialism in the Nineteenth Century* (New York: Oxford University Press, 1981).

colonial and Indian camps.[119] For example, the newly emerging educated middle class readily accepted western medicine since they perceived it as a benefit of the colonial government and associated its use as evidence of progress.[120] Similarly, Mark Harrison disagreed with the proposition that medicine was merely a 'tool of the Empire' and argued that it also displayed a humanitarian concern.[121] Jane Buckingham echoed Harrison's view in her work on leprosy asylums in colonial south India, arguing that medical institutions reflected the government's humanitarian concern.[122] However, Mridula Ramanna argued that while the government felt 'obliged' to provide public health facilities, 'financial discipline' limited such concerns.[123] While it is important to evaluate colonial motivations, the central objective of this project is not to ascertain colonial motivations for the establishment of asylum institutions. The primary aim of this book is to account for the Indian experience of the asylum and to evaluate the impact of the colonial asylum on Indian society.

Existing historical works provide some understanding of insanity, colonial psychiatry, and the asylum system of this period. However, several questions remain unanswered. In particular, these questions relate to local responses, traditional and local systems, and the agency of families. This study journeys through the nineteenth- and early twentieth-century Bombay Presidency, exploring some of these issues. The relationship and interaction between Indian communities and the asylum system as a colonial institution will remain its primary focus.

Scope and Significance

This book is a social history that locates itself within the historiographies of colonial medicine, psychiatry, and institutions. The work particularly seeks to highlight the experiences of patients and the local community as they

[119] David Arnold, *Colonizing the Body: State Medicine and Epidemic Disease in Nineteenth-Century India* (Berkley and California: University of California Press, 1993), pp. 288–289.

[120] Ibid., p. 241.

[121] Mark Harrison, *Public Health in British India: Anglo Indian Preventive Medicine, 1859–1914* (Melbourne: Cambridge University Press, 1994), pp. 228–230.

[122] Jane Buckingham, *Leprosy in Colonial South India Medicine and Confinement* (Basingstoke: Palgrave Macmillan, 2002), p. 4.

[123] Mridula Ramanna, 'Gauging Indian Responses to Western Medicine: Hospitals and Dispensaries, Bombay Presidency, 1900–1920', in Deepak Kumar (ed.), *Disease and Medicine in India: A Historical Review* (New Delhi: Tulika Books, 2001), p. 245.

encountered a colonial medical institution. An analysis of such experiences requires the right understanding of the local-colonial concept of mental health. This study therefore adopts Sudhir Kakar's definition of mental health: 'a label which covers different perspectives and concerns, such as the absence of incapacitating symptoms, integration of psychological functioning, effective conduct of personal and social life, feelings of spiritual and ethical wellbeing and so on'.[124] This definition differs from the western biomedical understanding that insists on a mind–body dualism and excludes the spiritual. For indigenous communities, the lack of the spiritual dimension in the healing process made asylums irrelevant. Such cultural difference caused colonial agencies to contend and undermine local mental health systems and health practitioners who they perceived as superstitious.

This study, in examining the lunatic asylum and its implications on local communities, presents and answers several interconnected questions. In doing so, this study has asked one main research question: What were the factors that led to the failure of the asylum system as a colonial institution in the Bombay Presidency? By using this question as a lynchpin, this study proceeds to explore other related aspects of the relationship between the asylum and local communities. First, the book examines the Indian perception of mental illness and traditional methods of dealing with madness. It then questions the impact of the coming of the asylum on local methods of dealing with the mentally ill. Next, it examines the nature of the asylum system and its implications in a colonial context. It closely reviews the fragmented asylum bureaucracy and ruptured relations among colonial agencies. The book further examines treatment methods used in Bombay's asylums. By analysing treatment methods from 1793 to 1921, the study points to the unchanging nature of treatment practices throughout this period. These treatment methods explain why the local community did not perceive the institution as a hospital.

Apart from ineffective treatment methods, even the asylum soundscape bears evidence of the failure of the asylum. This book is the first to explore the soundscape of Indian lunatic asylums. The term 'soundscape' is used both literally and figuratively to understand a paradox in Bombay's asylums. Bombay's asylums featured one of the most unruly soundscapes. Yet, at the same time, patients experienced 'epistemic violence'.[125]

---

[124] Kakar, *Shamans, Mystics and Doctors*, p. 3.

[125] Gayatri Spivak, 'Can the Subaltern Speak?', in Cary Nelson and Lawrence Grossberg (eds.), *Marxism and the Interpretation of Culture* (London: Macmillan, 1988), p. 24.

The study raises questions on the silencing and manipulation of patients' voices in the asylum. Finally, it raises questions about public perceptions of the lunatic asylum and the impact such perceptions had on the use and disuse of the asylum.

The study, in framing its chronological scope, deviates from the usual method of using lunacy legislation as a chronological reference point. A major point of difference between India and Britain, regarding the development of the asylum system, is the role of legislation. Legislation in Britain had a significant impact on the development of the asylum system. For example, the Asylums Act of 1808 enabled magistrates to establish county institutions. This Act led to the building of 13 county asylums between 1808 and 1834. Even with the implementation of the Poor Law Act of 1834 that categorized the mentally ill into two classes of 'idiots' and 'lunatics', the asylum population rose steadily. By 1837, the total patient population in new county asylums stood at 7000. The passing of the Asylums Act of 1845 only increased the asylum population, since it included 'idiots and imbeciles' as eligible for admission to an asylum. The following years saw a significant increase in the number of asylums and patients. By 1847, 36 of the 52 counties built their own asylums.[126] By 1850, five years after the passing of the Act, county asylums experienced overcrowding, with the total asylum population doubling to 15,000.[127] Lunacy legislation played a crucial role in facilitating the asylum movement in Britain.

By contrast, in India, legislation had little impact on the development of asylums. The two laws passed concerning lunacy during the period of this study were the Lunacy Act of 1858 and the Lunacy Act of 1912. Most historians of colonial psychiatry have generally tended to analyse colonial asylums in two distinct periods. The first period covers the asylum system under the East India Company (EIC); the second extends from the Queen's Proclamation and the passing of the Lunacy Act in 1858 to the Lunacy Act of 1912. Scholars take the year 1858 as a watershed to examine the expansion of the asylum system, based on the assumption that lunacy legislation propelled an era of asylum expansion. However, lunacy legislation failed to have a significant impact on the expansion of the asylum system in Bombay. Financial expediency was the most important

---

[126] Scull, *Museums of Madness*, p. 186.

[127] David Wright, 'Learning Disability and the New Poor Law in England, 1834–1867', *Disability and Society*, Vol. 15, No. 5, 2000, pp. 734–736.

factor influencing lunacy administration. In Bombay, public philanthropy rather than legislation, led to the building of the asylums after 1858. Moreover, several *mofussil* asylums existed prior to the passing of the Lunacy Acts of 1858 (as noted in Chap. 3). Furthermore, by examining the history of lunatic asylums in the Bombay Presidency from 1793 until 1921, this book seeks to demonstrate a continuity in the custodial character of asylums in Bombay. The change of power from the EIC to the Crown and the passing of the Lunacy Acts of 1858 and 1912 had little impact on the running of the colonial asylum. Proposed plans for improvement were greatly limited by meagre funding.

In terms of its conceptual framework, this research fits within the context of Edward Said's theory of Orientalism.[128] Said argued that the Orient was a 'body of theory and practice' that was essentially constructed by the West; this constructed 'system of knowledge' reinforced European superiority.[129] The field of mental health bears evidence of similar constructions of Indian knowledge and people. As argued in this book, the establishment of the asylum necessitated the construction of a narrative of Indians as 'stagnant' and 'superstitious'. Indian practice and knowledge of mental health treatment were rooted in an integrated spiritual-somatic understanding of insanity. However, colonial agencies projected Indian society as having an exclusive spiritual and therefore a 'superstitious' approach towards mental health. The construction of a narrative of the Indian population as stagnant and superstitious served to justify the necessity of the asylum and propagate its use. Even in independent India, the NMHP in 1982 unconsciously reiterated the belief in a superstitious Indian society; it emphasized the need for creating an awareness of mental illness in Indian society. What it essentially entailed was the creation of an awareness in local communities of a western-based epistemology of mental illness in an attempt to popularize the use of mental hospitals.[130]

METHODOLOGY AND SOURCES

This study primarily used the archival method of data collection in constructing its narrative. Primary sources including colonial records, some vernacular newspapers, and a few Indian sources (including a patient's

---

[128] Edward Said, *Orientalism* (New York: Vintage, 1979).
[129] Said, *Orientalism*, p. 14.
[130] National Mental Health Program, India, 1982, pp. 1–2.

letter) were analysed. The MSA and the National Archives of India (NAI), New Delhi, served as the main repository of primary sources. Apart from government consultations, the study has used Reports on Native Newspapers (RNP) to access vernacular newspapers. Additionally, India Office Records (IOR) at the British Library (BL), London, provided further evidence for this research. Digitized copies of Annual Asylum Reports made available by the National Library of Scotland (NLS) added to the evidence. The website www.archive.org was another repository used to access digitized nineteenth- and early twentieth-century books. The Heras Institute, Mumbai, also provided some primary materials like the Triennial Report for Civil Hospital and Dispensaries in the Bombay Presidency.

While the written records are fascinating, they have their limitations. One of the major defects in the colonial asylum archive on Bombay is the existence of several chronological gaps in existing accounts; often there are several stretches where the only records available are one-page reports of asylum visitors confirming that they were satisfied with the condition and management of the asylum. It is another reason why the book uses a thematic rather than chronological approach in its analysis. Second, the absence of patient registers and case notes and the meagre amount of patient and family letters are a serious drawback. This absence particularly limits the scope of the narrative, especially concerning women. This scarcity contrasts with Britain and colonies like Australia and New Zealand where a vast number of primary sources written by patients and their families relating to the asylum are available. Thus, the task of presenting a balanced colonial-local history is particularly challenging for historians of colonial asylums in India, as they must rely largely on government and asylum records, with few written accounts of patients or their families. Third, often certain terms are loosely used. For example, in the annual asylum records 'Caste' features alongside the religious categories of Hindu, Muslim, and Christians.

Another major drawback of the MSA is that the authorities concerned have destroyed several records. The archives only had documents until the year 1933. Records after 1933 were supposed to be available at the respective mental hospitals.[131] However, on my visit to Thana Mental Hospital, the staff told me that after a conflict with the archives over the storage of the files, the hospital burnt them due to lack of space. At the Ratnagiri

---

[131] Historians James Mills and Shruti Kapila have used these records in their research.

Mental Hospital, there were no such records either, except records of the recent years. My final visit was to the Yerawada Mental Hospital, Poona. Here, the superintendent did not grant me access to records or permission to take photographs on suspicion that I might be a journalist. My visit to the three main mental hospitals in 2014, nevertheless, provided interesting insights to the project. Photographs taken at the hospitals at Thana and Ratnagiri corroborated information collected at the archives.

CHAPTER OVERVIEW

The book is divided into five major themes (Chaps. 2, 3, 4, 5 and 6). The second chapter presents a brief history of Indian perceptions and treatment of mental illness from ancient times to the colonial period. Local communities adhered to an integrated spiritual-somatic approach towards insanity. This approach was rooted in Indian religious philosophy. For example, Vedic literature offered an understanding of the interconnected spiritual-somatic nature of human personality consisting of three elements. The first element is *aja* (similar to the concept of *aatman*, which is the essence of the indwelling universal force); the second element is *tanu* (likeness or shape, which includes the mind or *manas*); and the third is the *sarira* (the physiological organism).[132] Islamic philosophy holds a similar understanding of the human personality. A human being is not merely a physical being but contains *ruh* or the spirit of God and *nah* or the self (soul).[133] This chapter argues that the establishment of the asylums necessitated a colonial construction of the Indian understanding of mental illness and its treatment as entirely spiritual and consequently 'superstitious'. Colonial agencies used this narrative to justify the establishment of the asylum and promote its use. Along with asserting the superiority of western medicine, they undermined local agencies that traditionally provided treatment and care to those who suffered from mental illness. Furthermore, the chapter contends that the asylum, which was a response to Victorian society's capitalist–individualistic ideals, remained peripheral to the lifeworlds of Indian communities that were essentially collectivistic in nature.

---

[132] Karel Werner, 'Indian Concepts of Human Personality in Relation to the Doctrine of the Soul', *The Journal of the Royal Asiatic Society of Great Britain and Ireland*, Vol. 1, No. 1, 1988, pp. 77–78.

[133] Baltabayeva Alyonaa, Gabitov Tursunb, Maldubek Akmarala, Shamakhay Sairab, 'Spiritual Understanding of Human Rights in Muslim Culture' (The problem of "Ruh" – "Spirit"), *Procedia – Social and Behavioural Sciences*, No. 217, 2016, p. 714.

What appeared to be 'native apathy' towards the asylum system was indeed a response to the colonial misunderstanding of its spiritual-somatic conceptions of insanity and its collectivistic structure. Faced with apathy from local communities, the European superintendent struggled to attract them to the use of the asylums. By the early twentieth century, Bombay's colonial asylum system had become a failed colonial enterprise. Indian apathy was only one reason for the failure of this 'veritable Cinderella' in the family of colonial institutions.

The third chapter examines the power relations between the asylum bureaucracy and the role of a highly fragmented colonial official hierarchy as a cause of the failure of the asylum system between 1793 and 1921. This chapter argues that internal power contestations paved the way for negotiations with local people and their ideas, and this transformed Bombay's colonial asylum into a 'middle ground'.[134] Using the agency of superintendents as the lynchpin, the chapter examines the complex relationships and encounters between colonialism and Indians as they contested, resisted, and co-existed with each other. The creation of the asylum as a 'middle ground' in the colony meant that while some form of control was executed over patients, colonial hegemony was never complete.

The fourth chapter analyses the failure of the colonial asylum system through a study of its treatment methods. Superintendents in Bombay adopted the 'common-sense' treatment of Indian insanity that entailed hybrid treatment methods. Treatment methods in Bombay from 1793 to 1921 essentially revolved around clothing, feeding, and occupying patients. The chapter contends that such treatment methods based on preconceived notions of Indians were often culturally insensitive. These treatment practices often led to greater abuse of patients, since there were no boundaries about what constituted moral treatment.

The fifth chapter looks at the asylum soundscape for evidence of the failure of the asylum as a colonial medical enterprise. The chapter analyses the soundscape from 1814 to 1921. It begins in 1814, the year for which archives have the earliest surviving case notes of Assistant Surgeon J.A. Maxwell. The poorly regulated and regimented asylum soundscape is evidence that proves the custodial rather than curative character of Bombay's lunatic asylums. Most often, the poor regulation of sound was a result of financial constraints. While asylum agencies poorly regulated

---

[134] Richard White, *The Middle Ground: Indians, Empires, and Republics in the Great Lakes Region, 1650–1815* (Cambridge: Cambridge University Press, 1991).

noise, they manipulated patients' voices to serve the diagnostic process. Patients' voices also had evidential value, as asylum staff called upon them to act as witnesses in cases of staff neglect or deaths of other patients. However, government authorities and staff considered their evidence as 'reliable' only if it facilitated the continued agency of the superintendent. The control executed over patients' voices within the asylum also extended beyond asylum walls.

The sixth chapter analyses public perceptions of the asylum system and the influence that image had on its use by local communities. The chapter focuses on the period 1850–1921 and examines the perceptions of three Indian groups: the elite, the press, and the masses. The interest of the elite in the asylum was restricted to merely funding it for the sake of furthering their own interests. They perceived the asylum to be a place for the poor and destitute. The vernacular press exposed the asylum scandals, complaining of the ill treatment of patients within the asylum. The press played an important role in constructing the image of the asylum as a place of confinement. Local communities avoided the asylum since they deemed it as a punitive custodial institution, rather than one that provided medical treatment.

The concluding chapter provides an overview of the main research findings. This book, then, by analysing the internal and external factors associated with the lunatic asylum argues that the historical traumas associated with the asylum elicited Indian aversion to the asylum. These traumas disrupted the assimilation of the colonial lunatic asylum and ensured its failure as a colonial medical enterprise. Traumas in the Indian experience included the colonial undermining of Indian worldviews, cultures, practitioners, and patients. Additionally, the use of patients for labour and profit and epistemic violence within the asylum caused deep-seated historical trauma. Families also experienced trauma because of the stigma associated with the use of the asylum and the admission process. The aversion of the local community towards the asylum was a type of everyday resistance, a form of 'self -help'[135]—a defence mechanism to avoid being wounded further.

---

[135] James Scott, *Weapons of the Weak: Everyday Forms of Peasant Resistance* (New Haven: Yale University Press, 1985), p. 29, in Douglas Haynes and Gyan Prakash (eds.), *Resistance and Everyday Social Relations in South Asia* (Delhi: Oxford University Press, 1991), pp. 9–10.

CHAPTER 2

Indian Insanity and the Local-Colonial Contest for its Treatment

Nine years after the annexation of Sindh, the government began discussing plans to establish a lunatic asylum for the province. The Civil Surgeon of Sindh reported:

> To show that the natives of the Province have no objection either to confinement or medical treatment, we may mention that there is a private Establishment kept by a *Faqueer*[1] at Tigr near Serrsry in the Shikharpoor Collectorate where about 5–6 lunatics are always under the *Faqueer's* care and treatment.[2]

The Civil Surgeon inferred that local communities had no objection to 'confinement' or 'medical treatment' of their mentally ill relatives. Based on the information of the Civil Surgeon, the asylum system should have met with great success after its establishment. By 1912, however, superintendents reported that the poor response of local communities to the asylum system. Superintendent Overbeck-Wright pointed out that 'the people of India [had] an innate objection to sending their relatives to an

---

[1] *Faqueer* is the same as *fakir* (religious mendicant).
[2] From the Superintending Surgeon and Staff Surgeon, Sindh, to the Commissioner of Sindh, Kurachee, 24 June 1851, GoB, GD, 1852/10, MSA, Mumbai.

© The Author(s) 2018
S. A. Pinto, *Lunatic Asylums in Colonial Bombay*,
Mental Health in Historical Perspective,
https://doi.org/10.1007/978-3-319-94244-5_2

asylum for treatment'.[3] The response of Indian communities starkly contrasted the response of local communities in Britain, who depended on the asylum for the care of their mentally ill people.

In the context of the rise of the asylum in Britain, scholars have argued that there were intrinsic links between the invention of the asylum system and the evolution of ideas of insanity. The understanding of madness evolved from being a demonical manifestation[4] to a disease. People with mental illness, who were earlier labelled as 'lunatics', 'unfeeling brutes', and 'ferocious animals' in need of shackling were now perceived as 'sick human beings' in need of treatment and care.[5] Over the centuries, the increasing secularization of insanity in Britain gave mad-doctors their legitimacy as 'experts' of insanity, and asylums their legitimacy as medical institutions.[6] The expansion of the British Empire in the nineteenth century involved the exportation and proliferation of British institutions.

Medical institutions, along with jails and schools became an integral part of the colonial landscape.[7] Once the British established political hegemony in India, British colonists began ordering the empire through the establishment of institutions. Such institutions, as David Arnold argued, played an important role in 'socializing the masses into quiescent consent'. Medicine was an extension of the hegemonic agenda of the Raj and a 'benevolent counterpart to the coercive aspect of colonial rule'.[8]

When the British established the first lunatic asylum in Bombay in the late eighteenth century, local ideas of insanity and systems that provided care, treatment, and confinement for the mentally ill contested its agency. In India, traditional healers and community members adhered to an integrated spiritual-medical approach practised since ancient times. This approach was rooted in Indian religious philosophy. For example, in Vedic tradition, there is an intrinsic understanding of the interconnected

[3] A.W. Overbeck-Wright, *Mental Derangements in India: Its Symptoms and Treatment* (Calcutta and Simla: Thacker, Spink and Co., 1912), p. 101.

[4] Judith Neaman, *Suggestions of the Devil: The Origins of Madness* (New York: Anchor Press, 1975), p. 55.

[5] Elaine Showalter, *The Female Malady* (New York: Pantheon Books, 1985), p. 8.

[6] Andrew Scull, 'From Madness to Mental Illness: Medical Men as Moral Entrepreneurs', *European Journal of Sociology*, Vol. 16, No. 2, 1975, p. 254.

[7] Waltraud Ernst, *Mad Tales from the Raj: Colonial Psychiatry in South Asia, 1800–58* (New York: Anthem Press, 2010), p. 49.

[8] David Arnold, 'Public Health and Public Power: Medicine and Hegemony in Colonial India', in Daglar Engles and Shula Marks (eds.), *Contesting Colonial Hegemony: State and Society in Africa and India* (London, New York: British Academic Press, 1994), pp. 134, 139.

spiritual-somatic nature of humans that consists of three elements. The first element is *aja* (similar to the concept of *aatman*, which is the essence of the indwelling universal force); the second element is *tanu* (likeness or shape that included the mind or *manas*); and the third is the *sarira* (the physiological organism).[9] Islamic philosophy holds a similar spiritual-somatic concept of humans: a person is more than just a physical being, consisting of *ruh* or the spirit of God and *nah* or the self (soul).[10] This spiritual-somatic understanding translated into spiritual-somatic approaches to mental health treatment as elaborated in this chapter.[11] This chapter argues, then, that the establishment of lunatic asylums, necessitated a colonial construction of the Indian understanding of mental illness and its treatment as exclusively spiritual and consequently 'superstitious'.

The contradictions in beliefs and treatment approaches to mental illness led to a contention between traditional healers and the colonizers during the early nineteenth century. By the second half of the nineteenth century, the colonists targeted traditional health practitioners and care providers. Colonial agencies perceived the knowledge of traditional health practitioners as a threat to the justification of the civilizing mission. They then constructed a narrative of traditional health systems as 'stagnant' and 'superstitious', to establish the supremacy of western psychiatry and propagate the use of the asylum system. Such narrative is a classic example of what Nicholas Dirks termed the 'reconstruction and transformation' of Indian knowledge.[12]

This chapter argues that the establishment of the asylum system contended with Indian medical practices and belief systems. Colonial agencies consciously attempted to dismantle traditional health systems and marginalize traditional health practitioners because of the competition they posed

[9] Karel Werner, 'Indian Concepts of Human Personality in Relation to the Doctrine of the Soul', *The Journal of the Royal Asiatic Society of Great Britain and Ireland*, Vol. 1, No. 1, 1988, pp. 77–78.

[10] Baltabayeva Alyonaa, Gabitov Tursunb, Maldubek Akmarala, Shamakhay Sairab, 'Spiritual Understanding of Human Rights in Muslim Culture (The problem of "Ruh" – "Spirit")', *Procedia – Social and Behavioural Sciences*, No. 217, 2016, p. 714; Also see Sudhir Kakar, *Shamans, Mystics and Doctors* (Chicago: The University of Chicago Press, 1982), pp. 227–228.

[11] The intellectual unrest in nineteenth-century Maharashtra displays similar views on the links between science and spirituality or reason and faith, where 'Indian rationality remained amicably allied with spirituality'. See Hulas Singh, *Rise of Reason: Intellectual History of 19th-century Maharashtra* (New York: Routledge, 2016), p. 169.

[12] Nicholas Dirks, 'Foreword', in Bernard Cohn, *Colonialism and its Forms of Knowledge* (New Jersey: Princeton University Press, 1996), p. ix.

to western medicine. Despite British disapproval, however, local communities continued to use Indian treatment methods.[13] Ideological differences between the colonial and the local regarding insanity and its treatment failed to reconcile. The colonial state thus established the asylum in an ideological setting hostile to its growth.

Furthermore, the growth of asylums in Britain was directly linked to the restructuring of society based on 'capitalist market-principles',[14] which changed the nature of British societies into more individualistic societies. In such societies, productivity and profitability determined an individual's value. While not all families in Britain were willing to institutionalize their relatives, over the nineteenth century they increasingly used the asylum both as a place for 'short-term committal' and 'long-term care'. The decision of families and communities, as Cathy Smith argued, significantly determined asylum population, which increased at an alarming rate over the nineteenth century.[15] There were exceptions in the dichotomy of the collective and individual ideals presented between families in Britain and India and both sides were susceptible to class concerns. In comparison, however, Indian families or the community adhered to a more collectivistic value system, taking responsibility for the care of their mentally ill relatives. For Indian communities, the asylum system was irrelevant and peripheral as a means of treatment.

This chapter contends that the asylum as an institution failed because it challenged two important aspects of Indian society: first, the notion of an integrated spiritual-medical approach practised for centuries; and second, the community-centric nature of Indian society. The Alienist Department, the 'system of asylums and mental hospitals "established" or "licensed" by the Provincial Governments for the treatment of mental disorders under the Indian Lunacy Act of 1912',[16] thus doubly alienated itself and failed to assimilate into Indian society.

[13] Poonam Bala, '"Nationalizing" Medicine: The Changing Paradigm of Ayurveda in British India', in Poonam Bala (ed.), *Contesting Colonial Authority: Medicine and Indigenous Responses in Nineteenth and Twentieth Century India* (Lanham, Boulder, New York, Toronto, Plymouth: Lexington Books, 2012), p. 3.

[14] Andrew Scull, *Museums of Madness: The Social Organization of Insanity in Nineteenth-Century England* (London: Trinity Press, 1979), pp. 15, 48.

[15] Cathy Smith-Northampton, 'Family, Community and the Victorian Asylum: a Case Study of the Northampton General Lunatic Asylum and its Pauper Lunatics', *Family & Community History*, Vol. 2, No. 2, 1 November 2006, p. 122.

[16] W.S. Jagoe Shaw, 'The Alienist Department of India', *British Journal of Psychiatry*, Vol. 78, April 1932, p. 331.

INDIAN IDEAS OF INSANITY AND TREATMENT PRACTICES: ANCIENT TO COLONIAL INDIA

The discourse on the meanings of madness in Indian society existed since the Vedic times (3600–3000 BCE).[17] In Indian tradition, there were two meanings of mental illness. First, Indian society perceived mental illness as a disease of the mind, which traditional medicine could cure. Second, Indian society conceived of mental illness as a spiritual or supernatural phenomenon. Practitioners of traditional medicine and local communities inferred that these two meanings were interconnected at times and independent at other times. The *Atharvaveda,* the 'oldest medical book of the Hindoos', a book of incantations and spells (1200–1000 BCE), contains the earliest reference to insanity in ancient India.[18] It exemplified the interconnected approach towards insanity in Indian society:

1. Unbind and loose for me this man, O Agni, who bound and well restrained is chattering folly
   Afterward, he will offer thee thy portion when he hath been delivered from his madness.
2. Let Agni gently soothe thy mind when fierce excitement troubles it
   Well-skilled I make a medicine that thou no longer mayst be mad.
3. Insane through sin against the Gods, or maddened by a demon power.
   Well-skilled I make a medicine to free thee from insanity.
4. May the Apsarases release, Indra and Bhaga let thee go.
   May all the Gods deliver thee that thou no longer mayst be mad.[19]

The first step in the treatment process involved restraining the person, following which the *atharvan*[20] or 'sorcerer-priest'[21] administered medicine to the

---

[17] K.C. Singhal and Roshan Gupta, *The Ancient History of India, Vedic Period: A New Interpretation* (New Delhi: Atlantic Publishers and Distributors, 2003), p. 20.

[18] Sir Bhagavat Simhaji, *A Short History of Aryan Medical Science,* 1865–1944 (London, New York: Macmillan and Co., 1896), p. 25; Michael Witzel, 'Early Sanskritization: Origins and Development of the Kuru State', *Electronic Journal of Vedic Studies (EJVS),* Vol.1, No. 4, 1995, p. 4.

[19] *Hymns of the Atharva-Veda,* trans. Ralph T.H. Griffith (London: Luzac and Co., 1895), p. 306.

[20] Paul Masson-Oursel, Helena de Willman-Grabowska, Philippe Stern, *Ancient India and Indian Civilization,* trans. M. R. Dobie (London: Kegan Paul, Trench, Trubner & Co., 1951), p. 234.

[21] Ibid.

mentally ill person. Since madness was attributed to 'sin against the gods'[22] or to demonic possession, the *atharvan* simultaneously recited prayers.

In the Ayurvedic tradition, the treatment for the cure of insanity was called *Bhoot Vidya*. The prescribed treatment was 'prayers, offerings and medicine'.[23] Ancient Indian society ascribed to the notion that God was the 'first divine physician'. *Brahma*[24] himself gave the healing art of Ayurveda.[25] Medical knowledge and spiritual knowledge in India intertwined because the Hindus believed that God revealed all knowledge, including that of medicine and disease.[26] While the treatment approaches and understanding of mental illness found in the Vedas are not representative of the views of all Indian communities, it proves that India had a written tradition of a discourse on mental health since ancient times. The *Charakha Samhita* (1000 BCE), another ancient Indian medical book, also provides an elaborate discourse on insanity.

The book prescribed both an interconnected and an independent spiritual-somatic approach in the treatment of insanity.[27] The *Charakha Samhita* defined the symptoms of *Unmada* (insanity/insane) as 'wandering about of mind, intellect and consciousness, knowledge, memory, inclination, manners, activities and conduct'.[28] It attributed mental illness to 'Non-Exogenous and Exogenous factors'. Non-Exogenous factors included eating 'deficient', 'cold', 'uncooked' food and 'pungent, sour, burning or hot edibles', 'Excessive saturation', 'slow activity', 'excessive evacuation', fasting and 'wasting of *dhatus*'.[29] Exogenous insanity was caused by evil spirits, gods, ancestors, *gandharvas* (celestial being known to cause possession and ecstasy),[30] *yaksa* (spirit or demi-god), *raksasa* (demon), *brahmaraksasa* (ghost of a Brahman who led an unholy life or a demon), and *picasa* (demon). The book suggests that insanity caused by possession by god and *gandharvas* was positive, apart from the usual symptoms of loss of sleep and appetite. An excessive desire for worship, music, and dance that was accompanied by an auspicious smell was

[22] Ibid.
[23] Simhaji, *A Short History of Aryan Medical Science*, p. 25.
[24] In the Hindu tradition, Brahma is God who is the creator.
[25] Simhaji, *A Short History of Aryan Medical Science*, p. 25.
[26] Ibid., p. 24.
[27] Singhal and Gupta, *The Ancient History of India*, p. 3.
[28] Gabriel Van Loon (ed.), *Charakha Samhita: Handbook on Ayurveda*, Vol II. (New Delhi: Chaukhambha Orientalia Publishers, 2002), p. 1100.
[29] *Dhatus* are the seven tissues of the body: plasma, blood, muscle, fat, bone, marrow/nerve and reproductive tissue; https://www.ayurvedacollege.com/articles/drhalpern/the-seven-dhatus-tissues-ayurveda; accessed 8 October 2016.
[30] M. Monier Williams, *A Sanskrit-English Dictionary* (Delhi: Motilala Banarassidas Publishers, 2005), p. 346.

characteristic of insanity caused by gods or *gandharvas*. Those displaying such symptoms were treatable through the recommended measures. Madness attributed to *raksasas, brahmaraksasas* and *yaksas, picasas*, ancestors, and other evil spirits, however, had no positive attributes; it often led to self-destructive and violent behaviour. The book deemed violent insanity in which a person showed suicidal tendencies to be incurable.

While Indian society attributed madness to spirit possession, it also believed that an individual held responsibility for his own madness in certain cases. The *Charakha Samhita* condemned the implication of 'the gods, forefathers or *raksasas* of a disease caused by one's own deeds through intellectual error'.[31] Intellectual errors included disregarding gods or demons, and other religious figures, or rebelling against the authority of parents or teachers. Insanity was also a result of bad actions or sinful actions from one's past life.[32] A person's intellectual error led to madness, since it opened the door to the infliction of madness upon one's self by gods, demons, and spirits. The *Charakha Samhita* listed steps for preventing madness caused by intellectual error. Measures recommended included having a *sattwa*[33] nature, abstinence from meat and wine, having a wholesome diet, and being sincere and pure.[34]

Treatment in ancient India was a combination of medicine and mantra. The physician had to determine the cause and type of insanity, based on which he administered treatment.[35] Therapy for curable insanity included 'unction, fomentation, emesis, purgation, non-unctuous and unctuous enema, pacification, snuffing and smoking, fumigation, inhalation of herbal juice, blowing (into nose), massage, paste, bath, striking, tying, confinement, frightening, inducing surprise, desaturation and bloodletting, proper dietic regimen according to *dosas* (bodily humors)'.[36] While confinement was a part of therapy, the *Charakha Samhita* recommended

[31] Van Loon, *Charakha Samhita*, p. 1108.
[32] Ibid., p.1103.
[33] 'The Indian scriptures, particularly the *Samkhya* books and the *Bhagavad Gita*, classified *Gunas* (traits/natures) into *sattwa, rajas*, and *tama*.' *Sattwa Guna* entailed 'purity, serenity, humility, forgiveness, transparency, compassion, altruism, contentment, dispassion'. *Rajas Guna* incorporates 'Greed, jealousy, impatience, pride, suspiciousness, vindictiveness, anger'. *Tama Guna* is characterized as 'ignorance, inertia, forgetfulness, negligence, laziness, procrastination'. See S. Elankumaran, 'Personality, Organizational Climate and Job Involvement: An Empirical Study', *Journal of Human Values*, Vol. 10, No. 2, October 2004, p. 119.
[34] Van Loon, *Charakha Samhita*, pp. 1106–1107, 1116.
[35] Van Loon, *Charakha Samhita*, p. 1116.
[36] Ibid., p. 1102.

it only for unsubmissive patients. In such cases, soft bandages served to restrain the patient who was then kept in an isolated room. Apart from these, *Charakha Samhita* prescribed a combination of traditional drugs. In the case of insanity caused by gods, the book instructed physicians to avoid 'harsh measures' and use only mild medicaments and various rituals and prayers. It also suggested the worship of the Hindu god Shiva for freedom from the fear of insanity and the god Rudra for the cure of insanity.[37] The association between the spiritual and somatic understanding of insanity continued into the medieval era.

In medieval Indian society, families took primary responsibility for their relatives suffering from mental illness. Regarding medical systems, the coming of the Unani (Muslim school of medicine) during this period enriched Indian medical traditions.[38] The story of the mystic Mirabai (1498–1557) provides insight into the way families managed madness. Mirabai was a medieval Indian princess who adopted an unconventional way of life and broke traditional norms of behaviour. She renounced her husband and royal life because of her devotion and relentless passion for Krishna, the Hindu god.[39] Most people, including her own family, disapproving of her behaviour labelled her a lunatic.[40] Mira's family attempted to change her behaviour using several methods that ranged from binding her to giving her medicines and even an alleged attempt to murder her.[41] Indian families tried to manage mentally ill relatives within their domestic confines. If they failed to manage the person, they resorted to local doctors, healers, and caretakers. In Mira's case, her 'madness' was first treated with rebuke and ridicule. Her family members used dissuasion to correct madness. They rebuked and ridiculed the person's behaviour to shame the person out of their 'madness' or unconventional behaviour. Mira's 'madness' provoked her husband's fury, her mother in law's taunts, and her sister-in-law's teasing.[42] While Mira was aware that her family was trying to

[37] Ibid., p. 1116.

[38] Sanjeev Jain, 'Psychiatry and Confinement in India', in Roy Porter and David Wright (eds.), *The Confinement of the Insane: International Perspectives, 1800–1965* (New York: Cambridge University Press, 2003), pp. 273–274.

[39] *Mirabai −54 Poems-*, Classic Poetry Series, 'Torn in Shreds', 2012, p. 53; www.poemhunter.com; accessed 14 July 2015.

[40] *Mirabai −54 Poems-*, 'Mine is the Lifter of Mountains and Mira Danced with Ankle Bells', pp. 31, 33.

[41] Ibid., 'Mine is the Lifter of Mountains', p. 31.

[42] *Mirabai −54 Poems-*, 'Mine is the Lifter of Mountains, p. 31.

discipline her, she also noted her mother-in-law's empathy. In one instance, she wrote of how her mother-in-law wept while trying to restrain her.[43]

When words of rebuke or ridicule failed, the family used other methods to manage her mental illness. Mira's family physically restrained her and kept her confined in a room.[44] The failure of physical restraint to correct madness led to the family seeking external help for treatment. The family called a traditional doctor who administered medicines for the cure of insanity to treat Mira's 'madness'. Mira recounted in her poems that the *Vaidya* (doctor) forcefully administered medicines to her. When the doctor failed to cure her 'madness', Mira alleged that her brother-in-law tried to murder her for disregarding the family honour.[45] Mira left home and wandered about. Mira's madness now confronted the local community. Society's response to Mira's 'madness' was a mixture of ridicule and reverence. Mira recalled that 'some point[ed] fingers at her'[46] and 'some praised her devotion'.[47] While some of those deemed mentally ill wandered about in society, there were also instances of hospitals for confinement and treatment.

Historical evidence points to the existence of a few hospitals for treating mentally ill persons during this period. Shridhar Sharma noted that there were 'asylums' during the reign of Mohammad Khilji (1296–1316) and a hospital under the management of Maulana Fazulur Hakim in Madhya Pradesh.[48] Hospitalization for mentally ill persons, however, was the exception rather than the rule. Medieval Indian society managed madness mostly within the confines of the family and in some cases with the help of spiritual healers and traditional doctors.

In the nineteenth century, medieval Indian society upheld the integrated spiritual-somatic understanding of insanity and its corresponding treatment methods. For Indian communities, the asylum system established in Bombay in 1793[49] would remain peripheral to the care of those suffering from mental illness. European superintendents complained that among Indian families the 'unhappy creatures' were 'concealed in Private

---

[43] Ibid., 'I Write of that Journey', p. 24.
[44] Ibid, 'Friend without the Dark Raptor', p. 14.
[45] *Mirabai – 54 Poems*, p. 3.
[46] Ibid., 'No One Knows my Invisible Life', p. 35.
[47] Ibid., 'Torn in Shreds', pp. 31–33.
[48] Shridhar Sharma and L.P. Varma, 'History of Mental Hospitals in the Indian Sub-Continent', *Indian Journal of Psychiatry*, Vol. 26, No. 4, 1984, p. 295.
[49] From Civil Architect [to Bombay Castle], 7 November 1793, GoB, Public Department Diary (PDD), 1793, No. 107, Part 1, MSA.

parts of the House in order to conceal their family misfortune and to remove them from Harm's way'.[50] Home remedies included incensing the person, waving eggs or limes around their face, and fulfilling any vows that the family of individual made to the gods.[51] When medicine failed, families attributed mental illness to spirit possession. The Hindus would usually call a Brahmin who would 'drive the spirit away' by reading from the Vedas and Puranas.[52] The Muslims would call a *Syed*, a holy man to administer incense-ashes and holy water and occasionally perform an exorcism on the person.

Exorcists consisted of two classes: professional and non-professional. The former learnt exorcism from a teacher; the latter claimed inspiration from spirits. Local communities referred to exorcists by different names. Hindus referred to them as *devrishis* or divine seers, *mantris* or enchanters, *bhagats* or devotees, and *panchakharis*[53] and the Muslims called them *vastads* or teachers. Exorcists were both men and women. Exorcists used both religious methods and local medicines. The Hindu exorcist mostly employed incantations, incensing, charmed ashes, healing herbs, amulets, and paper with the names of Hindu gods. Animals and food were part of the offering to the demon or god possessing the person. In an exorcism, the exorcist also used water infused with leaves of the Indian birch tree. The Muslim exorcist would use talismans, recitation of the name of Allah, and fumigation. A thread called *nadapudi* was tied on the wrist or neck of the person suffering from mental illness; it was used both by Hindu and Muslim exorcists. If the exorcist failed to cure the person, the family took them to shrines of different deities. In the Bombay Presidency, the four most popular shrines were Narsobas Vadi in Kolhapur, Alandi and Narsingpur in Poona, Phaltan in Satara, and Gangapur near Sholapur.[54] The Muslims took their relatives who suffered from mental illness to Sirvada or Karadgaon where there were tombs of their saints. In Gujrat, the Mira Data Dargah, a shrine dedicated to Mohemedan Pir was 'visited

[50] From the Civil Surgeon, Dharwar, to Simson Esquire, 3 August 1844, GoB, GD, 1844/34/380, MSA.

[51] James Campbell (ed.), *Gazetteer of the Bombay Presidency: Poona*, Part 1 (Bombay: Government Central Press, 1885), p. 555.

[52] James Campbell, 'Notes on the Spirit Basis of Belief and Customs', *Indian Antiquary*, Vol. 23, December 1894, p. 379.

[53] *Panchakharis* were exorcists who chanted the *panchakshari* mantra during exorcism. See Govind Narayan, *Mumbai: An Urban Biography from 1863*, trans. Murali Ranganathan (New York: Anthem Press, 2009), p. 267.

[54] Campbell, *Gazetteers of the Bombay Presidency: Poona*, p. 559.

by many suffering from epilepsy'.[55] At the shrines or tombs, the person who suffered from mental illness had to serve in the temple, worship the idol, and bring offerings to the gods or ascetics.[56]

Of the various local practitioners providing treatment for mental illness, *fakirs* were commonly associated with the confinement, care, and treatment of mentally ill people. The *Gazetteer of the Bombay Presidency: Poona* described *fakirs* as those who provided mystical chants or spells to 'non-professional exorcists'.[57] While primarily an ascetic, a *fakir* did not restrict himself to spiritual matters. In Hyderabad, a *fakir* operated a 'private Establishment' to look after people suffering from mental illness. Even the Civil Surgeon at Hyderabad acknowledged that the *fakir* administered 'medical treatment' to the 'lunatics' under his care.[58] In Punjab, *fakirs* maintained a shrine that cared for microcephaly sufferers. The local name for such people was Shah Daula's *chuas* (mice), because of their 'flattened skull' and 'prominent ears'.[59] Major George Ewens, Superintendent of the Punjab Lunatic Asylum, described the place as 'practically an asylum' where they were 'tended and cared for until their death'. He also observed that local communities had no objection to the shrine; in fact, it was 'well known, and its premises were always open to inspection'.[60] *Fakirs* and *sadhus* (ascetics) administered a juice made of indigenous herbs for the 'cure of insanity'.[61] Indian communities had their own systems of care, custody, and treatment for mentally ill people.

These traditional systems provided competition to the asylum and its doctors. Indian knowledge of mental health treatment and its practitioners

---

[55] F.A.H. Elliot (ed.), *Gazetteer of the Bombay Presidency: Baroda*, Vol. VII (Bombay: Government Central Press, 1883), p. 619.

[56] James Campbell (ed.), *Gazetteer of the Bombay Presidency: Kolhapur District*, Vol. 24 (Bombay: Government Central Press, 1886), p. 420.

[57] Campbell, *Gazetteers of the Bombay Presidency: Poona*, p. 555.

[58] From the Superintending Surgeon and Staff Surgeon to the Commissioner of Sindh, Kurachee, 24 June 1851, GoB, GD, 1852/10, MSA.

[59] Overbeck-Wright, *Mental Derangements in India*, pp. 99–100.

[60] George Ewens, 'An Account of a Race of Idiots Found in the Punjab, Commonly Known as "Shah Daula's Mice", *Indian Medical Gazette*, Vol. 38, 1903, pp. 330–334, in M. Miles (ed.), Disability Care and Education in 19th Century India: Dates, Places and Documentation with Some Additional Material on Mental Retardation and Physical Disabilities, Document Type: Information Analyses, US Department of Education, May 1997, pp. 25–26.

[61] Annual Report on the Working of the Ranchi Indian Mental Hospital, Kanke in Bihar for the Year 1936, p. 12, NLS.

put the British colonists in a dilemma. They had to acknowledge India's rich oral and written traditions of medical knowledge. In Africa, it was easier to undermine indigenous knowledge, which largely existed in the form of oral traditions. It was convenient to label the African as 'primitive' and 'savage' in the absence of written sources. In India, however, the evidence of the existence of a civilization and its written and oral knowledge traditions necessitated the writing of a new narrative of local peoples.[62] This new colonial narrative led to the subversion of traditional medical knowledge and health practitioners by assigning labels of 'stagnant' and 'superstitious' to them.

COLONIAL NARRATIVE OF INDIAN IDEAS OF INSANITY AND TREATMENT PRACTICES

The establishment of lunatic asylums necessitated the construction of a new narrative to justify the institution and promote its use. This colonial narrative was used as evidence for the 'stagnated' and 'superstitious' character of Indian society. Furthermore, this narrative was essential for the justification of colonialism, based on the 'European Idiom' of bringing the fruits of 'progress and modernity'.[63] In the context of mental health, this implied the asylum system. The colonial narrative portrayed Indian communities as having an exclusive spiritual approach towards the treatment of mental illness. Colonial agencies constructed this narrative in three phases. The first phase was the observation and collection of information on the traditional treatment practices of Indians. The second was the disparaging of traditional knowledge, and the third was the undermining of Indian health practitioners. Despite colonial attempts to disrupt Indian health systems, local communities continued to use them for treating their mentally ill relatives.

In the early nineteenth century, the practice of observation and collection of information of Indian health systems resulted in the publication of books on local medical practices. Published works of European travellers aided in the process of gathering information about Indian medical

---

[62] Ashish Nandy, *The Intimate Enemy: Loss and Recovery of Self Under Colonialism* (Delhi: Oxford University Press, 1983), p. 17.

[63] Michael Mann, 'Torchbearers Upon the Path of Progress: Britain's Ideology of Moral and Material Progress in India', in Harald Fischer-Tiné and Michael Mann (eds.), *Colonialism as Civilising Mission*, (London: Anthem Press, 2003), p. 5.

systems. Fra Paolino Bartholomeo, a Carmelite missionary and Austrian professor of Oriental languages in Rome, wrote *A Voyage to the East Indies* in 1796. After having travelled in India for 13 years, he recorded in his book his observations of places 'little frequented by the Europeans'.[64] On the medical knowledge of India, he wrote, 'India alone contains more medical writings, perhaps than are to be found in the rest of the world'.[65] He also praised the local Malabar physicians as 'more superior than most Europeans in knowledge of the Simples [simple medicine]'.[66] The French traveller Pierre Sonneret's views on Indian medical system juxtapose with Bartholomeo's views. Sonneret suggested that 'Indians [were] mostly pretenders to some knowledge of medicine'. The English doctor Ainslie Whitelaw, however, dismissed Sonneret's view as untrue.[67]

At the onset of colonial rule in India, European physicians served as surveyors. One such surveyor was Dr. Ainslie Whitelaw. In 1813, he wrote *Materia Medica*. A second edition of the book, published in 1827, was a treatise on Indian drugs and health remedies. The *Medico-Chirurgical Review*, a British medical journal, in its review of the book, praised it for providing information of 'native remedies employed by Hindoos ... [and] modes of employing them', since the British were 'entirely in the dark' about these local remedies.[68] The *Monthly Review* appraised the *Materia Medica* for removing, undoubtedly, 'any prejudice ... about the advanced stage of Hindoo knowledge about the subject of medicine'.[69] Works published during this period created a new awareness of the effectiveness and advancement of Indian treatment practices, despite its antiquity. The *Medico-Chirurgical* also added in its review that Ayurveda

> was adapted to the limited faculties of man, and consisted of eight divisions ... the fourth [*Bhoot Vidya*] was the treatment of mental derangement (**so that the ancient Hindoos had *mad doctors* as well as the modern European**).[70]

---

[64] *The Monthly Review*, May–August, Vol. XXXII, 1800, p. 237.

[65] Fra Bartholomeo, *A Voyage to the East Indies*, trans. William Johnson (London: J Davies, 1800), p. 412.

[66] Bartholomeo, *A Voyage to the East Indies*, p. 413.

[67] Ainslie Whitelaw, *Materia Medica of Hindoostan, and Artisan's and Agriculturist's Nomenclature* (Madras: Government Press, 1813), p. 64.

[68] *Medico-Chirurgical Review and Journal of Practical Medicine*, New Series, Vol. 6 (London: G Hayden, 1827), p. 397.

[69] *The Monthly Review*, Vol. 5, May–August 1827, p. 142.

[70] *Medico-Chirurgical Review*, p. 406. Text in bold for emphasis.

Colonial observation and collection of Indian medical knowledge clearly pointed to an expansive storehouse of medical knowledge available in India. The *Materia Medica* elaborated that the 'the articles used by the Hindoos in Medicine are extremely numerous, much more so than any Materia Medica in Europe'.[71] Colonial observers, however, found it hard to accept the fact that an interwoven spiritual-medical system was effective in India and that its practitioners were 'highly venerated'.[72] Once colonial agencies gathered information on the Indian methods of the treatment of insanity, they interpreted this knowledge to serve the process of disparaging local treatment practice and practitioners.

Since western psychiatry itself was still in its nascent stages, colonial agencies had little evidence to argue for the superiority of western knowledge regarding the treatment of insanity. In Bombay's asylums, confinement and treatment of physical symptoms remained the chief treatment for insanity. As Dr. W. Campbell, Superintendent of the Colaba Lunatic Asylum elaborated:

> What is done in the way of medical treatment may be summarily told in a single sentence. It consists in attention to health and the removal or alleviation, as far as possible of any bodily disease.[73]

Confronted with the failure to present an alternative narrative of a 'scientific' and 'superior' treatment of insanity, colonists began writing a counter-narrative which presented Indian treatment practices as purely spiritual and therefore 'stagnant' and 'superstitious'. The new narrative served as the first step in dismantling Indian medical knowledge systems.

Colonial observers published records that described 'spirit possession' as the most widely attributed cause of insanity in local communities. The *Gazetteer of the Bombay Presidency: Kolhapur District*

---

[71] Ainslie Whitelaw, *Materia Indica; or, Some Account of those Articles which are Employed by the Hindoos and Other Eastern nations, in Their Medicine, Arts, and Agriculture: Comprising also Formulae, with Practical Observations, Names of Diseases in Various Eastern Languages, and a Copious List of Oriental Books Immediately Connected with General Science, &c.* (London: Longman, Rees, Orme, Brown and Green, 1826), p. xxxiv.

[72] Ibid., p. xiii.

[73] From the Superintendent, Colaba Lunatic Asylum, to the Secretary to the Principal Inspector General, Medical Department, 31 July 1863, GoB, GD, 1862–1864/15, MSA.

documented that among local communities in the Deccan, irrespective of their religion,[74]

> a patient is believed to be possessed by an evil spirit if his eyes are bloodshot or bleared as if with drink, if he suffers from shooting pains, if he keeps crying or weeping, if he talks too much, does not speak for days or answers questions with abuse, if he refuses food for days or eats too much and yet feels hungry, if he lets his hair fall loose, and sways his body to and fro, if he faints, suffers from cramps, or spits blood.[75]

Colonial publications served to reinforce preconceived colonial stereotypes of local peoples. Even Hemp Commissioners[76] noted:

> ignorant and uneducated persons ascribe[d] a child's epilepsy to his having accidentally touched the painted stone that represents the village god, while playing under the sacred tree, or a fit of insanity to an attack or possession of a *Bhut* or village Ghost ... who believe in no cause which they do not see, except witchcraft, whose powers of observation are quite unexercised and undeveloped.[77]

James Campbell, a British official, in his 1894 article titled 'Notes on the Spirit Basis of Belief and Customs', elaborated how Indian society adhered to the belief that 'all diseases were caused by spirits'.[78] In a similar vein, S.M. Edwardes, the Commissioner of the Bombay Police wrote

---

[74] The *Gazetteer of Poona* also provides a similar description: 'In the Deccan if a person cries or weeps incessantly, if he speaks at random, if he sways his body to and fro, if he lets his hair fall loose, if he spits blood, if he does not speak or if he refuses his food for several days, and grows day by day paler and leaner, he is believed to be possessed by a spirit'. See Campbell, *Gazetteer of the Bombay Presidency: Poona*, p. 553.

[75] Campbell, *Gazetteer of the Bombay Presidency: Kolhapur District*, p. 415.

[76] The Hemp Drugs Commission was set up in 1893 in 'response to the questions raised in the British Parliament'. The commission aimed to conduct an enquiry into the Indian use of hemp in order to regulate its use. The enquiry was intended to primarily focus on hemp use in Bengal, but it was extended to the whole of India. It consisted of 'written and oral examination of 1193 witnesses' who included 'civil and medical officers, European and native medical practitioners, farmers, traders and missionaries' and hemp users. See Oriana Kalant, 'Report of the Indian Hemp Drugs Commission, 1893–94: A Critical Review', *The International Journal of the Addictions*, Vol. 7, No.1, 1972, pp. 77–78.

[77] Report of the Indian Hemp Drugs Commission, 1894–1895, Vol. 2, p. 232, NLS, Scotland.

[78] *Indian Antiquary*, p. 374.

By-ways of Bombay, a book describing the local community, especially its approaches to illness. The book contained pictures that depicted how the local community dealt with mental illness. One example is the picture of the Possession of Afiza (Fig. 2.1). Edwardes records the story of Abdullah the *dhobi* (laundry man) who believed that a spirit had possessed his wife after childbirth. The picture depicts Abdullah, his wife, mother, and the *Syed* exorcising the spirit from Afiza.[79] Such publications served to provide evidence for the construction of a narrative of Indian society as stagnant and superstitious. The colonial construction of a narrative that Indian ideas of insanity and its treatment were purely based on spiritual beliefs served to legitimize their claims of the 'white man's burden' to administer 'scientific' treatment of mental illness through the asylum system.

By the mid-nineteenth century, colonial agencies felt so threatened by local treatment systems that they considered their repression essential to maintaining 'colonial order'.[80] Colonial agencies consciously targeted local health practitioners and those who provided treatment for the mentally ill. They labelled these practitioners as either 'lunatics' or 'quacks'. Catharine Coleborne identified a similar concern among colonial authorities in New Zealand about 'quackery and superstition' among the Maori, which led to a prosecution of Tohunga (experts), accused of using 'illegal' medical practices.[81] Likewise, in Zululand, Julie Parle argued that missionaries accused 'native incantators' of causing 'indiki'[82] possessions and charging a 'fee...for curing it'.[83] In the Bombay Presidency, over the nineteenth century, an increasing number of *fakirs* and religious mendicants found themselves incarcerated. In 1903, Superintendent Ewens accused the *fakirs* who looked after the microcephalic sufferers in Punjab of 'neglect and ill treatment', while, oddly, noting that the local community had no objections to the shrine. By 1912, the practice of the *fakirs* taking the persons suffering from microcephaly begging was 'practically put to a

[79] S.M. Edwardes, *By-ways of Bombay* (Bombay: D.B. Taraporevala and Sons, 1912), pp. 52–56.

[80] Gyan Prakash, *Another Reason: Science and the Imagination of Modern India* (New Jersey: Princeton University Press, 1999), p. 129.

[81] Catharine Coleborne, *Madness in the Family: Insanity and Institutions in the Australasian Colonial World, 1860–1914* (Manchester: Palgrave Macmillan, 2010), p. 62.

[82] In Southern African beliefs, indiki is a spirit that causes possession in men and women. See Julie Parle, 'Witchcraft or Madness? The Amandiki of Zululand, 1894–1914', *Journal of Southern African Studies*, Vol 29, No. 1, March 2003, pp. 105–132.

[83] Ibid., p. 110.

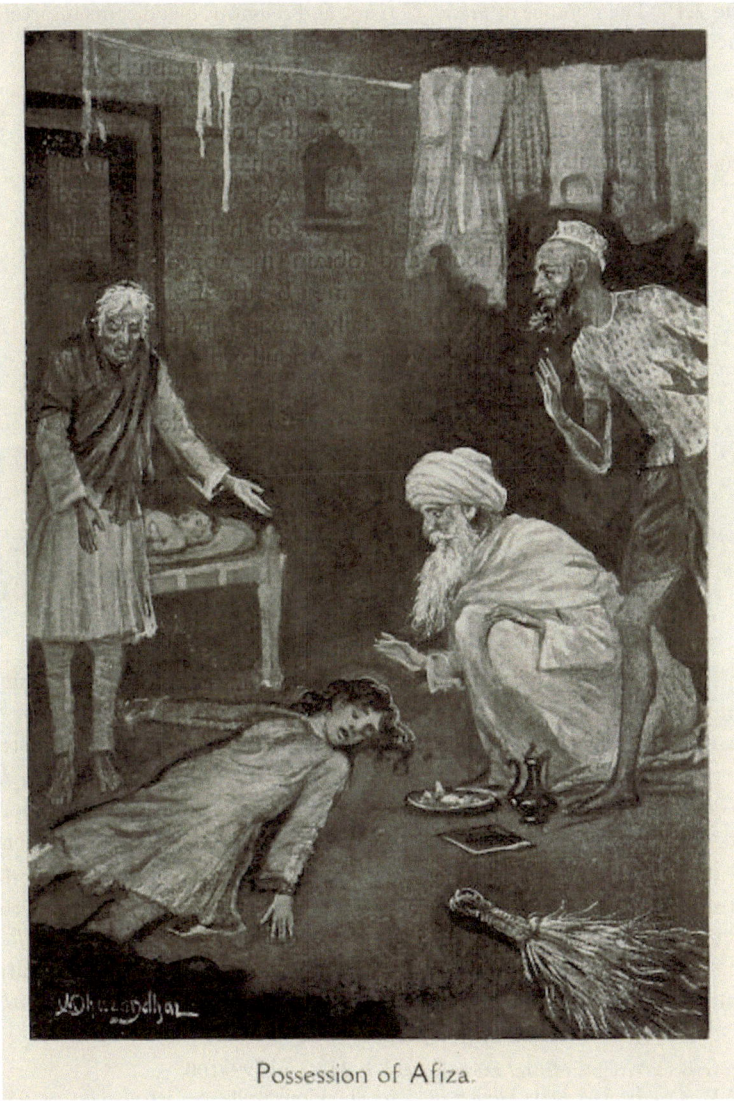

Possession of Afiza.

Fig. 2.1 *Possession of Afiza*, a picture in the book *By-ways of Bombay*. (Source: S.M. Edwardes, *By-ways of Bombay* (Bombay: D.B. Taraporevala and Sons, 1912), p. 55)

Table 2.1   The number of *fakirs*, beggars, and religious mendicants incarcerated in the Asylums of the Bombay Presidency (1876–1900)

Year	Beggars, religious mendicants, and fakirs[a]	Total patient population
1879	50	260
1880	60	230
1881	50	237
1882	54	304
1883	58	329
1884	46	315
1885	46	315
1886	47	265
1887	47	242
1888	48	265
1889	34	242
1896	61	292
1897	39	190
1899	20	303

[a]After 1900 the word *fakir* is no longer mentioned in Annual Asylum reports of the Bombay Presidency

Source: APR, 1879, p. 12; APR, 1880, p. 12; APR, 1881, p. 2; APR, 1882, p. 2; APR, 1883, p. 12; APR, 1884, p. 12; APR, 1885, p. 12; APR, 1886, p. 14; APR, 1887, p. 12; APR, 1888, p. 10; APR, 1889, p. 12; APR, 1896, p. 16; APR, 1897, p. 16; APR, 1899, p. 20; NLS

stop'.[84] The practice, however, continued, notwithstanding attempts by colonial authorities to restrict the *fakirs*.[85]

Authorities labelled the class that made provision for the care, custody, and treatment of Indian mentally ill people as 'lunatics'. The *Medical Jurisprudence of India* elaborated that the masses held 'religious mendicants' like 'sadhus and fakirs' in 'reverence'; however, they were 'certifiably insane' and 'extremely dangerous'.[86] In 1850, the Civil Surgeon of Ahmedabad explained that 'all devotees and ascetics, when not imposters, suffer to some extent from insanity'.[87] Between 1876 and 1900, *fakirs* along with beggars and religious mendicants formed the largest patient population in Bombay's asylums. Table 2.1 depicts the number of *fakirs*,

[84] Overbeck-Wright, *Mental Derangements in India*, pp. 99–100.

[85] A.W. Overbeck-Wright, *Lunacy in India* (London: Bailliere, Tindall and Cox, 1921), pp. 179–180.

[86] Lyon Isidore Bernadotte, *Medical Jurisprudence for India, with Illustrative Cases*, Vol. 7(Calcutta: Thacker and Spink, 1921), pp. 353–354.

[87] From the Superintending Surgeon to the Magistrate, Ahmedabad, 16 August 1849, GoB, GD, 1850/51, MSA.

beggars, and mendicants incarcerated in Bombay's lunatic asylum for this period.[88] While they formed the largest group in the patient population, doctors also perceived them as suffering from more serious or incurable types of insanity. *Fakirs* as patients, explained Dr. Overbeck-Wright, were in such a deplorable condition when admitted, that they 'got their identities lost beyond their recovery'.[89] In the Annual Reports for 1897–1899, as seen in Table 2.1, there was a sharp drop in the number of *fakirs* incarcerated. A strange shift appears in Annual Asylum Reports after 1900. The Reports no longer use the word *fakir* in categorizing patients. One could speculate that this change could mean that for colonial doctors *fakirs*, after this period, were akin to beggars and mendicants. While colonial authorities dealt with *fakirs* and religious mendicants by incarcerating them in asylums, they simultaneously began contesting the medical authority of *vaids* and *hakims*.

Colonial agencies used allegations of 'quackery' to undermine local medical practitioners, since local communities preferred them to the institution of asylum. The *Gazetteer of the Bombay Presidency, Poona*, 1885 categorized *Vaidus* (Vaidyas) as 'beggars'. It further elaborated that these physicians visited the Poona district annually to sell their 'drugs and medicines, and, under the pretense of working cures deceive[d] ignorant and simpleminded people'.[90] Superintendent J. Keith interviewed ex-patients and families in 1894 to gather information on the links between hemp use and insanity as part of the Hemp Commission Report. The family of an ex-patient, Metho, explained that they first took him to the 'native *hakim*'. In the published interviews with Metho's family and other patients, Surgeon Keith inserted the word 'quack' after 'native *Hakim*' when the family mentioned going to such a practitioner.[91] The Superintendent of the Central Lunatic Asylum at Yerawada described Indian treatment methods during the early twentieth century as a mixture of 'quack medicines and charms'.[92] Faced with competition from traditional practitioners claiming expertize on Indian insanity, colonial allegations of quackery

---

[88] The Annual Report in 1876 stated: 'Many fakirs and sepoys have been admitted'. APR 1876, p. 26, NLS; also see Table 2.1.

[89] Overbeck-Wright, *Lunacy in India*, p. 6.

[90] Campbell, *Gazetteer of the Bombay Presidency: Poona*, p. 477.

[91] Report of the Indian Hemp Drugs Commission, 1894–1895, Vol. 2, pp. 185, 189, NLS.

[92] From the Superintendent, Central Lunatic Asylum, Yerawada, to the Surgeon General with the Government of Bombay, 26 May 1922, GoB, GD, 1922/2257, MSA.

were a means of undermining traditional treatment methods. On one hand, colonial agencies accused Indian practitioners of quackery, on the other, they criticized them for 'keep[ing] their remedies a secret ... making research difficult, and limiting the spread of knowledge'.[93]

The Indian press had mixed responses to the colonial accusations of quackery among local medical practitioners. The *Yajdan Parasat* in 1871 recommended that the government should prohibit 'ignorant *Hakims* and *Vaidyas* from practising and licence only those who possess a good knowledge of country medicine and country practice'.[94] In 1880, when discussions began over a proposal put forward by the government to register medical practitioners, a vernacular newspaper contested the rights of local practitioners.[95] The *Native Opinion* advocated for local health practitioners, arguing that even though 'no allusion was made in the Bill prohibiting *vaids* and *hakims* from practising ... the fact that all registered practitioners must be those who practised European medicine' would act as a hindrance to the 'vocation' of *vaids* and *hakims*.[96] It also added that 'these classes of medical practitioners [who have] existed for ages, have been appreciated and still perform many useful functions'. In defence of the Indian medical tradition, the *Native Opinion* maintained that from the 'Old Hindu and Mohemedan books there is much to be learnt and that they contain many prescriptions which are cheap and suitable to the people and the climate'.[97]

Colonial endeavours to gain hegemony over Indian medical systems and notions of insanity continued into the early decades of the twentieth century. Dr. Overbeck-Wright in his book *Lunacy in India* recommended a 'prophylactic campaign'. The 'first and most important step' of prophylaxis was 'to uproot the old superstitions and prejudices regarding such cases and asylums'.[98] He also endorsed the establishment of an out-patient department connected to the asylum that would help in the 'dissemination of knowledge'.[99]

[93] Triennial Report on the Civil Hospitals and Dispensaries of the Bombay Presidency, 1923–1925 (Bombay: Government Central Press, 1927), p. 14.

[94] RNP), *Yajdan Parasat*, 25 April 1880, K 409, J–D 1880, PG 1–444, MSA.

[95] Mridula Ramanna, *Western Medicine and Public Health in Colonial Bombay, 1845–1895* (New Delhi: Orient Longman, 2002), p. 208.

[96] RNP, *Native Opinion*, 25 April 1880, K 409, J–D 1880, PG 1–444, GoB, MSA.

[97] RNP, *Native Opinion*, 25 April 1880, K 409, J–D 1880, PG 1–444, GoB, MSA.

[98] Overbeck-Wright, *Lunacy in India*, p. 137.

[99] Ibid., p. 138.

Such campaigns made colonial interference with local customs inevitable. Consequently, Indian communities were afraid of the European doctor's interference with their religious ceremonies. In 1912, S. M. Edwardes' *By-Ways of Bombay* recorded Indian customs, especially with respect to the treatment of physical and mental diseases. Edwardes observed that the Muslims of Bombay took their sick relatives to a *Syed* who cured them. *Syeds*, he observed, would also exorcise 'the spirit of hysteria that so often lays hold of young women'.[100] He also visited various local communities to observe their treatment of physical and mental illness. He recorded that the *Bhandaris*,[101] who knew 'little of the western theories of health and sanitation', held a bi-weekly ceremony to 'propitiate the cholera goddess'.[102] The *Bhandaris*, according to Edwardes, interpreted his presence in two ways: 'Some feared him as one that contemplated the imposition of a new tax, others viewed him as a doctor from the hospital dispatched by higher authority to put an end to the ceremony'.[103] Local communities resented European doctors for propagating western medicine through the disruption of local customs and practices.

Campaigns for uprooting 'superstitious' health practices and practitioners received a setback with the beginning of a religious revivalist movement in the 1920s.[104] The revivalist movement, rooted in a new awareness in Indian society that 'colonial policies [were] detrimental to Indian science and medicine',[105] challenged the colonial narrative on the nature of Indian medical knowledge. Superintendent J. Shaw complained that 'the noisy section of the population led by M. K. Gandhi prefers the Ayurvedic and other indigenous systems to our modern methods of treatment. These so-called "systems" are based on very primitive ideas of anatomy and physiology, and are even more out-of-date than that of Galen'.[106]

Constant interference with local socio-religious practices failed to change Indian perceptions on local healing traditions and western

---

[100] S.M. Edwardes, *By-ways of Bombay* (Bombay: D.B. Taraporevala and Sons, 1912), p. 81.

[101] A local community in colonial Bombay who mainly lived in Dadar and Mahim.

[102] Edwardes, *By-ways of Bombay*, p. 66.

[103] Edwardes, *By-ways of Bombay*, p. 73.

[104] Bala, '"Nationalizing" Medicine', p. 11.

[105] Ibid., pp. 3, 4.

[106] W.S. Jagoe Shaw, 'The Alienist Department of India', *British Journal of Psychiatry*, Vol. 78, April 1932, p. 334.

medicine. A government report on India in 1923 attributed the failure of public health policies to 'unpopularity' caused by interference in 'traditional habits and methods of livelihood'.[107] The colonial state continued to contest Indian social customs and observances, believing that Indians needed to be 'weaned from their tenacious adherence to social observances which [were] as diametrically opposed to public health as they are to economic prosperity'.[108] Indians, however, contested the colonial belief in the superiority of scientific treatment in an asylum. Even former asylum patients induced local communities to resort to 'incantations and saints' for the cure of their insanity.[109] The masses continued to revere local practitioners and fear the European doctor. The popular understanding of insanity as a medico-spiritual condition facilitated the continuance of Indian health care systems that provided such integrated methods of treatment.

The 'noisy masses' made the government reflect on its public health policies and its insistence on scientific medicine. The Triennial Report on Civil Hospitals and Dispensaries of 1925 contained a discussion of Indian systems of medicine. The report projected western medical science as not a 'purely European one'. Surgeon Hooton, Surgeon General of the Indian Medical Service (IMS), explained:

> The modern system incorporated many of the old remedies, and it is easy to substantiate the contention of the advocates of the indigenous systems that the methods of treatment which have been hailed as new discoveries of the modern school have their counterparts in the East long ago ... Modern scientific method should not be regarded with hostility as a stranger in India but welcomed as a younger branch of the same family.[110]

While asserting that modern western medicine was rooted in eastern medical traditions, the Surgeon General staunchly defended the superiority of western medicine. He credited the colonial state for reviving Indian medical tradition, noting that: 'The ancient wisdom has returned, reinforced by

---

[107] L.F. Rushbrook Williams, *India in 1923–24* (Calcutta: Government of India, 1924), p. 213.

[108] Ibid., p. 212.

[109] From the Asst. Surgeon, Colaba Lunatic Asylum to the Secretary of the Medical Board, Government of Bombay, 21 February 1847, GoB, GD, 1847/41, MSA.

[110] Triennial Report on the Civil Hospitals and Dispensaries of the Bombay Presidency, 1923–1925 (Bombay: Government Central Press, 1927), p. 14.

new ideas and new discoveries which make it many times more valuable'.[111] His claims fitted perfectly into the colonial belief that ancient Indian medical traditions had declined over time because of 'modern Hinduism' and its caste regulations.[112] The colonial state that consciously engaged in the dismantling of Indian medical practices now claimed to be its champion.

COMMUNITY-CENTRIC NATURE OF INDIAN SOCIETY

Indian societal and domestic structures rendered the colonial asylum inefficacious.[113] Indian society is community-centric in nature. David Mandelbaum rightly argued that in India 'a person's whole life experience is embedded in his family relationships'.[114] Such ideals of 'interconnection and interdependence' in India can be traced to the ancient belief of all life originating from one source. Since Brahma created everything, his essence or *aatman* dwells in everyone.[115] Indian families reflected these community-centric ideals by taking primary responsibility for the care of their relatives who suffered from mental illness. Like families, ideals of group loyalty and cohesiveness are also characteristic to communities in India.[116] In the context of mental health, this meant that the mentally ill persons were part of the community:

> In the village, a mental defective is considered as part and parcel not only of the family but also of the whole community. He has a sense of belonging resulting from his being accepted by the community for what he is.[117]

Indian family and societal structures were organized to facilitate the management of mental illness within the family and community. Similarly, in Africa, Edgar and Sapire argued that the management of mental illness by

[111] Triennial Report on the Civil Hospitals and Dispensaries of the Bombay Presidency, 1923–1925 (Bombay: Government Central Press, 1927), p. 14.

[112] *The Imperial Gazetteer of India: The Indian Empire, Administrative*, Vol. IV (Oxford: Clarendon Press, 1909), pp. 457–458.

[113] J.B.P. Sinha, *Psycho-Social Analysis of the Indian Mindset* (New Delhi, New York, Heidelberg, Dordrecht: Springer, 2014), p. 27.

[114] David Mandelbaum, *Society in India* (Berkley: University of California Press, 1970), p. 41.

[115] Sinha, *Psycho-Social Analysis of the Indian Mindset*, p. 29.

[116] Geert Hofstede, *Culture and Organizations: Software of the Mind* (London: McGraw Hill, 1991), p. 51.

[117] Extract from the Indian Conference of Social Work in J.A. Marfatia, 'Welfare of the Mentally Handicapped', in A.R. Wadia (ed.), *History and Philosophy of Social Work in India* (Bombay: Allied Publishers, 1961), p. 378.

the family and community were 'collective social responses to afflic-
tions'.[118] In India, colonial doctors perceived such collective ideals of
Indian families as an obstruction to the use of the asylum. Superintendent
Overbeck-Wright observed that the people of India had an 'innate objection to sending their sick relatives away from home'.[119]

Conversely, the growth of large asylums and the consequent segregation of the insane in England was a result of 'massive reorganisation of an
entire society along market principles'.[120] Before the rise of asylums in
Britain, families had other formal and informal ways of confining mentally
ill persons. As nation states attempted to centralize the government, they
also began to homogenize mental health policies across regional entities
and local communities and take responsibility for the care of the insane.
Asylums were the state's solution to the problem of insanity in societies
transformed by urbanization and industrialization.[121] For families, the asylum was an additional option for treatment. Over the nineteenth century,
the socio-economic values of families changed based on capitalist market
principles. This change made them more willing to admit 'idle or unproductive' relatives.[122] In such a society that prioritized self-interest, the
lunatic asylum based on the individualistic ideals of Victorian society
served to relieve families of the responsibility of their mentally ill relatives.
It also functioned as an institution that taught self-discipline to those
deemed mentally ill in order to make them productive.[123]

Colonial agencies, however, perceived Indian family structures as an
obstruction to productivity and self-discipline. They therefore undermined Indian family structures. They believed that Indian families were
the source of superstitious beliefs, and a hindrance to the progress of

[118] R. Edgar and H. Sapire, *African Apocalypse: The Story of Nontetha Nkwenkwe, a
Twentieth- Century South African Prophet* (Johannesburg: Witwatersrand University Press,
2000), p. 46 in Parle, 'Witchcraft or Madness?', p. 118.

[119] Overbeck-Wright, *Mental Derangements in India*, p. 101.

[120] Andrew Scull, *Museums of Madness: The Social Organization of Insanity in Nineteenth-
Century England* (London: Trinity Press, 1979), pp. 15, 48.

[121] Ibid., pp. 15, 44.

[122] Michel Foucault, trans. Richard Howard, *Madness and Civilization: a History of
Madness in the Age of Reason* (New York: Tavistock Publications, 1973) and Klaus Doerner,
Madmen and the Bourgeoisie: A Social History of Insanity and Psychiatry (Oxford: Blackwell
Publishers 1981) in David Wright, 'Getting Out of the Asylum: Understanding the
Confinement of the Insane in the Nineteenth Century', *Social History of Medicine*, Vol. 10,
No. 1, 1997, pp. 137–155.

[123] Scull, *Museums of Madness*, p. 72.

Indian society.[124] Moreover, they constructed the idea of a 'joint family' system. This joint or extended family system came to represent the community-centric ideals of Indian society. Colonialism constructed the joint family as the 'chief domain where oppressive and restrictive patriarchal control was exercised'.[125] A Report on India in 1923 criticized the joint family system:

> The Hindu joint family system prevails. This ancient venerable institution has many social advantages; but from the point of view of industrial progress, it is a depressing rather than an elevating factor. It tends to penalise the able and the industrious for the benefit of the lazy and the incompetent.[126]

Colonial agencies blamed the joint family system for encouraging laziness in 'incompetent' family members. British observers accused Indian families of supporting 'drones instead of workers'.[127] Through the asylum system, these 'incompetent' members would learn to internalize self-discipline. Colonial agencies projected capitalist-individualist values on to Indian families. The collectivistic nature of Indian society was evidently a hindrance to such a colonial enterprise.

The colonial state through the establishment of asylums endeavoured to change the community-focused character of Indian families and society because it contended with the 'material and highly individualised ideals of the Western World'.[128] Indian families, however, resisted and contested this change. Local communities chose to confine their mentally ill people behind 'bamboo and clay' walls of their homes, rather than 'brick and mortar' asylum walls.[129] Families petitioned for the release of their relatives even when a magistrate had certified them as 'criminal insane', or they petitioned for a transfer of their relatives to an asylum closer to home. Duri Mohamad, whose brother Ouzal was a criminal patient at the

---

[124]Leigh Denault, 'Partition and the Joint Family in the Nineteenth-Century North India', *The Indian Economic and Social History Review*, Vol. 46, No. 1, 2009, p. 29.

[125]Ibid., pp. 29–30.

[126]Williams, *India in 1923–24*, p. 196.

[127]Phear, Mr. Justice John Budd. 'The Hindoo Joint Family', A Lecture Delivered at the Bethune Society 18 March 1867', in The Proceedings and Transactions of the Bethune Society from 10 November 1859 to 20 April 1869, Calcutta, 1870, in Denault, 'Partition and the Joint Family', p. 34.

[128]Williams, *India in 1923–24*, p. 194.

[129]Report on the Lunatic Asylum at Colaba for the Year Ending 1852, GoB, GD, 1853/48, MSA.

Ratnagiri Asylum, petitioned the government to move his brother to an asylum closer to his native place.[130] Local communities resisted the labouring of patients in the asylum. A local newspaper objected to the practice of the Superintendent at the Colaba Asylum making patients carry provisions.[131] Indian families and the community in most cases resisted asylum agencies or acted with indifference.

The close family and community ties in India that led to a poor response towards asylum committals are in contrast to the attitudes and response of families in colonies like Australia. In Australia, families accepted the asylum system, since white settler 'families were not marked by strong ties'.[132] Among Maori families in New Zealand, however, a similar aversion existed to asylum use. Maori communities, like Indian communities, had strong community bonds. Their incarceration in asylums by colonial authorities displayed a lack of cultural understanding of the significance of 'collective identities for Maori themselves'.[133] Even in colonial Bombay, police authorities and magistrates had little empathy towards Indian collectivistic ideals as they sent Indians to the asylum. In fact, magistrates conducted the process of medical certification in open places in India, publicly stigmatizing not only the individual patient but also the family.[134] Therefore, their confinement within the home protected the sick individual and others from harm, and protected the family honour. The aversion of local families to the asylum indicated that there was a stigma attached to the process of asylum admission.

The colonial asylum thus tended to undermine traditional community-centric values and contended to replace them with more individualistic ideals. Such a colonial ideal of an Indian society based on market principles would serve to maximize colonial profits and induce self-discipline, since every member of society would work to achieve productivity. Local families, nevertheless, resisted this change as they continued to care for their mentally ill relatives and opted for traditional healing methods. The asylum system remained peripheral to their lives. Chapter 5 of this book fur-

---

[130] Government Resolution, JD, Bombay Castle, 27 March 1915, GoB, GD, 1915/336, MSA.

[131] RNP, *Akbari Sowdagar*, 13 April 1871, K 406, J–D, 1871, PG 1–543, GoB, MSA. The *Akbari Sowdagar* was a Gujarati weekly.

[132] Coleborne, *Madness in the Family*, p. 60.

[133] Ibid., p. 62.

[134] Bernadotte, *Medical Jurisprudence for India*, p. 407.

ther elaborates on the agency of Indian families and the community in response to the asylum.

CONCLUSION

The total number of patients in the lunatic asylums of the Bombay Presidency in 1905 stood at 1203, a trivial number in comparison to the asylum population of Britain where at least 'a[one]lakh' (100,000) patients were treated in Victorian asylums every year.[135] Faced with the challenge of establishing the superiority of western medicine, colonial observers constructed a narrative of Indian medical systems as stagnant and superstitious. Colonial agencies also consciously undermined Indian practitioners to facilitate the use of the asylum. Local communities, however, continued to use Indian mental health systems that reflected a connected spiritual-somatic approach to mental illness. Poor asylum admissions stood as a testament to a silent resistance to the colonial undermining of traditional medical systems and family structures. Asylum superintendents lamented this poor response from local communities. While colonial agencies outside asylum walls showed increasing intolerance towards local social customs and medical systems, behind asylum walls superintendents began to devise strategies to make its use more relevant to Indian communities. In the asylum, superintendents disrupted the process of hegemonization as they began negotiating with the local community to ensure the survival of the institution.

[135] RNP, *Bombay Samachar*, 5 June 1906, January to June (J–J), 1906, GoB, MSA.

CHAPTER 3

The Asylum as 'Middle Ground': Contestations and Negotiations

In 1896, the Home Department in its reply to the Hemps Commission Report noted that

> the defects [of the asylums] pointed out (by Fraser and Warden) were in a great measure attributable to four causes, the two chief of which were the existence of a system under which the charge of the lunatic asylums was usually a minor part of work of the Civil Surgeon instead of the duty of a full time officer, and the failure of medical officers, superior and subordinate to make a special study on Insanity.[1]

However, Superintendent J.P. Barry of the Colaba Lunatic Asylum had a different perspective about the failure of asylums:

> This branch of public service has been so starved as to make it the veritable Cinderella of the family … The conscience of the Government has never been smitten by the blow of a great mortality or a great scandal, and so all these long years the system, such as it is, was carried on in a spirit that

[1] From the Government of Bengal to the Home Department, Government of India, Administration of Lunatic Asylums in India, 25 August 1896, Medical Proceedings, Simla Records 4, Home Department Notes, 1897, Nos. 188–232, NAI, New Delhi.

Richard White, *The Middle Ground: Indians, Empires, and Republics in the Great Lakes Region, 1650–1815* (Cambridge: Cambridge University Press, 1991).

© The Author(s) 2018
S. A. Pinto, *Lunatic Asylums in Colonial Bombay*,
Mental Health in Historical Perspective,
https://doi.org/10.1007/978-3-319-94244-5_3

61

seemed to grudge everything except good food, and so our asylums have all
the poverty-stricken bareness of a barrack room or godown with no hospital
equipment, nurses, sick accommodation, special drugs, &c. To remedy all
this it is not enough to add another patch to the existing ones, but to take
up the whole matter in a large spirit and bring it under the rules of system
and common sense.[2]

The two statements exemplify the constant bickering between the colonial
state and the asylum medical class. The colonial state, displaying a clear lack
of accountability, conveniently blamed the medical class for the failure of
the asylum system. Denouncing the colonial state, Superintendent Barry
believed that the state was liable for the failure of the asylum system because
of its meagre funding and unprincipled planning towards lunacy administration. Other superintendents in the Presidency echoed similar views.[3] The
colonial state and the medical class, despite their differences about the liability for the failure of asylums, concurred that the asylum system had failed.

Foucault, in his analysis of states and power, argued that institutions must
be analysed from the standpoint of power relations. States depend on these
power relations to function effectively. The British Raj was the 'superstruc-
ture' to a 'whole series of power networks' dealing with the colonial subjects' 'body, sexuality ... family, kinship, knowledge, and technology'.[4] In
the case of the lunatic asylum, which worked as a power network, the power
relations between the asylum agencies and the judicial and penal department were crucial to its functioning. This chapter examines these power
relations within the asylum bureaucracy, and the role of a highly fragmented
colonial bureaucratic hierarchy as a cause of failure of the asylum system.
Internal power contestations created a distance between the colonial state
and asylum superintendents. The chapter argues that these power contestations paved the way for negotiations with the Indian staff, families, and
patients and transformed Bombay's colonial asylum into a 'middle ground'.[5]

[2] From Lt. Col. J.P. Barry, Superintendent, Colaba Lunatic Asylum, to the Personal Asst.
to the Surgeon General with the Government of Bombay, 25 June 1904, GoB, GD,
1907/81, MSA, Mumbai.

[3] From Lt. Col. J.P. Barry, Superintendent, Colaba Lunatic Asylum to the Personal Asst. to
the Surgeon General with the Government of Bombay, 25 June 1904, GoB, GD, 1907/81,
MSA.

[4] Michel Foucault, *Power/Knowledge: Selected Interviews and Other Writings, 1972–1977*
(New York: Pantheon, 1980), p. 122.

[5] White, *The Middle Ground*.

The chapter uses Richard White's concept of the 'middle ground'. White, in his analysis of American Indian–French relationships, brought to light the development of a 'common ground or middle ground' between the Algonquian and the French as their 'worlds' met. The middle ground existed because of the inability of both sides to 'gain their ends through force'. It survived through the establishment of 'common conventions' between the two sides.[6] As British and Indian worlds met in the asylum, the European Superintendent and Indian staff, families, and patients created 'common conventions' within the asylum to meet 'specific ends'. For example, superintendents gave in to demands of relatives for frequent visits. Such negotiations ensured the survival of the institution. Negotiations, however, affected the colonial 'hegemonic project'.[7]

The transformation of the asylum into a 'middle ground' interrupted the actualization of hegemony in the colonial asylum. Using Gramsci's definition of hegemony, David Arnold contended that medicine and public health were 'part of the hegemonic project' of the government.[8] It constituted an 'ideology thickly impregnated with British political ambitions'. Medicine played a significant role in persuading Indians of their need for the British and thus in legitimizing colonial rule.[9] Keeping in line with Arnold, this chapter uses Gramsci's concept of hegemony: the organization of society based on 'consent' of the masses: a 'consent', which is created by the power position of the ruling group.[10] In lunacy administration and asylum affairs, superintendents as colonial agents failed to 'create' consent as they negotiated with Indian staff, families, and patients. These negotiations resulted instead in the creation of the middle ground. These negotiations also meant that while asylum staff executed some form of control over the patients, they failed in actualizing colonial hegemony. Using the agency of superintendents as the focal point, the chapter examines the complex relationships and encounters between colonialism and the Indian population as they contested, resisted, and co-existed with each other.

---

[6] Ibid., pp. 51–51.

[7] David Arnold, 'Public Health and Public Power: Medicine and Hegemony in Colonial India', in Daglar Engles and Shula Marks (eds.), *Contesting Colonial Hegemony: State and Society in Africa and India* (London, New York: British Academic Press, 1994), p. 140.

[8] Arnold, 'Public Health and Public Power', p. 140.

[9] Ibid., p. 139.

[10] Antonio Gramsci, *Selections from Prison Notebooks* (New York: International Publishers, 1971), pp. 170, 263 in Arnold, 'Public Health and Public Power', p. 132.

BOMBAY'S BEWILDERED BUREAUCRACY

Colonialism thrived through the establishment of institutions. The government managed these institutions through the creation of hierarchies. The Indian colony consisted of the three presidencies (of Bombay, Calcutta, and Madras), six provinces, and a few dependent territories. Once the East India Company achieved political hegemony, it established medical institutions and services.[11] The Bombay government established a Hospital Board in the Presidency in 1787,[12] and in 1796 they rechristened it as the Medical Board. For 20 years since the establishment of the Bombay Hospital Board, it consisted of only two members.[13] The Medical Board came under the authority of the Governor and his Council. After the passing of the Queen's Proclamation in 1858, the Crown took over all services of the EIC. The IMS finally replaced the Medical Board in 1897.[14] The asylum hierarchy had the government at its pinnacle. The government assigned the monitoring of the system to the Medical Board and later to the IMS. A Director General headed the IMS and each presidency had its own Surgeon General.[15] With the transfer of power to the Crown in 1858, the government set up Bombay's Public Works Department (PWD)[16] and assigned it with the construction of asylum buildings.[17] However, its work was 'complicated since Supreme government kept financial direction'.[18] The Lunacy Act of 1858 established a committee of Visitors who were responsible for supervising the asylum system. The committee included officers from the penal, judicial and medical departments.[19] Police and magistrates facilitated the admission of

[11] Muhammad Umair Mushtaq, 'Public Health in British India: A Brief Account of the History of Medical Services and Disease Prevention in Colonial India', *Indian Journal Community Medicine*, Vol. 34, No. 1, January 2009, pp. 6–14.

[12] D.G. Crawford, *A History of the Indian Medical Service, 1600–1913* (London: W Thacker and Co., 1914), p. 25.

[13] Ibid., p. 33.

[14] Crawford, *A History of the Indian Medical Service*, p. 293.

[15] W.S. Jagoe Shaw, 'The Alienist Department of India', *British Journal of Psychiatry*, Vol. 78, April 1932, p. 336.

[16] S.M. Edwardes, 'District Administration in Bombay, 1858–1919', in H.D. Dodwell (ed.), *The Cambridge History of the British Empire, 1497–1858*, Vol. V1, 2nd Edition (London: Cambridge University Press, 1932), p. 263.

[17] Sir Wilson William Hunter, *Bombay 1885–1890: A Study in Indian Administration:* (London: H. Frowde; Bombay, B.M. Malabari, 1892), p. 316.

[18] Ibid., p. 275.

[19] Lunacy Act XXXVI of 1858, GoB, GD, 1862–64/15, MSA.

patients.[20] Superintendents relied mostly on Indian and a few European subordinate staff to manage the asylum.[21] Patients featured in the lowest rungs of the asylum hierarchy.[22] The policy of 'native agency and European superintendence' reiterated by the House of Commons in 1853 was at the heart of the colonial asylum system.[23]

In 1793, the East India Company laid the foundation of the asylum system in the Bombay Presidency when it sanctioned the first exclusive accommodation for mentally ill people.[24] A set of five apartments in the seaman's Barracks at Butcher's Island was constructed. Its walls were 'twenty-two inches thick and eighteen feet in heigh[t]' and its doors and windows were 'strongly secured with iron bars'. The government additionally sanctioned a separate set of rooms for necessary attendants and an assistant surgeon, instituting a new asylum hierarchy. The asylum was 'allotted by the government' for those 'patients in this unhappy situation [of insanity]'.[25] The government shifted the asylum on Butcher's Island in 1799/1800 to a 'private house owned by Surgeon R. Fildes' in Colaba.[26] In 1826, when the Bombay government opened a new asylum at Colaba, they closed the private house asylum. This asylum functioned as the main government asylum for the Presidency in the nineteenth century.

[20] From the Acting Clerk, Petty Sessions, to the Chief Secretary to the Government of Bombay, 14 June 1812, GoB, PDD, 1812/336, MSA.

[21] Amna Khalid, 'Subordinate Negotiations; Indigenous Staff, the Colonial State and Public Health', in Biswamoy Pati and Mark Harrison (eds.), *The Social History of Health and Medicine in Colonial India* (New York: Routledge, 2009), p. 45.

[22] Shilpi Rajpal, 'Colonial Psychiatry in Mid-Nineteenth Century India: The James Clark Enquiry', *South Asia Research*, 2015, Vol. 35, No. 1, p. 75.

[23] Verney Lovett, 'The Development of the Services, 1858–1918', in H.D. Dodwell (ed.), *The Cambridge History of the British Empire, 1497–1858*, Vol. VI, 2nd Edition (London: Cambridge University Press, 1932), p. 362.

[24] Crawford stated that the earliest mention of lunatic asylums in the Presidency was in the consultations of 14 March 1745/46 ordering a place to be built for lunatics. See D.G. Crawford, *A History of the Indian Medical Service, 1600–1913*, Vol. 2, pp. 395, 400. In 1793, the Civil Architect petitioned the building of the asylum on Butcher's Island, noting that 'there was no such convenience [facility to maintain lunatics] earlier'. From the Civil Architect (to Bombay Castle), 7 November 1793, GoB, PDD, 1793/107, Part 1, MSA.

[25] Lunacy Certificate issued by Surgeon Scott for Benjamin Robertson, 11 July 1797, Bombay Castle, GoB, PDD, 1797/126, MSA.

[26] Waltraud Ernst, 'Racial, Social and Cultural Factors in the Development of a Colonial Institution: The Bombay Lunatic Asylum (1670–1858)', *Internationales Asienforum*, Vol. 22, No. 3–4, 1991, p. 64.

The establishment of asylums in the Bombay Presidency happened in a rather haphazard and slow manner. During the first half of the nineteenth century in most parts of the *mofussil*, civil hospitals had insane hospitals attached to them.[27] The insane hospital at Poona established in 1823[28] was a 'make-shift' arrangement, since it was originally a private dwelling house. The Surgeon General reported it as ill-suited for treating patients.[29] The earliest reference to an 'insane hospital' in Ahmedabad was in 1849.[30] An insane hospital attached to the civil hospital at Surat also treated patients. In 1863, authorities transferred patients from Surat and Ahmedabad to the new asylum at Ahmedabad.[31] Deliberations for opening an asylum in Dharwar started in 1845[32] and the government opened a new asylum there in 1851.[33] The British annexed Sindh in 1843. For administrative purposes, they included Sindh as part of the Bombay Presidency. The government established the first asylum in Sindh at Larkana in November 1861. The asylum was an old fort belonging to the Kalhora dynasty. In 1871, using the donation of Sir Cowasji Jehangir, the government built a new asylum in Hyderabad.[34] The *Gazetteer of Kolhapur* records a lunatic asylum attached to the civil hospital at Kolhapur that treated 37 patients in 1883–1884.[35] The last asylum built in the closing decades of the century was the Ratnagiri Asylum, established in 1886.[36] In 1902, a new asylum

[27] A government letter notes that there were asylums in Sholapur and Karachi. The 'asylum' at Sholapur consisted of a few cells attached to the civil hospital. From the Director General of the Medical Department with remarks form the Inspector General of Prisons, 9 December 1858, GoB, GD, 1859/24, MSA.

[28] APR, 1874–1875, p. 15, NLS, Scotland.

[29] APR, 1874–1875, p. 15, NLS.

[30] From the Bombay Medical Board Office to the Secretary to the Government of Bombay, 8 February 1850, GoB, GD, 1849/38, MSA.

[31] From the Principal Inspector General, Medical Department, to the Secretary to the Government of Bombay, 18 June 1863, GoB, GD, 1862–64/15, MSA.

[32] From the Superintending Surgeon to the Secretary of the Medical Board, Belgaum, 15 March 1845, Medical Department, GoB, GD, 1845/43/949, MSA.

[33] From the Chief Engineer, PWD, to the Governor and President in Council, 1 September 1851, GoB, GD, 1851/15, MSA. Up till 1850, patients from Dharwar were sent to the Colaba Lunatic Asylum. Medical Board Report, Bombay Castle, 15 May 1850, GoB, GD, 1850/51, MSA.

[34] A.W. Hughes, *A Gazetteer of the Province of Sindh* (London: George Bell and Sons, 1874), pp. 490–491.

[35] James Campbell (ed.), *Gazetteer of the Bombay Presidency. Kolhapur District*, Vol. 24 (Bombay: Government Central Press, 1886), p. 288.

[36] From the Cooks(Raghoo and Pandoo), Ratnagiri Lunatic Asylum, to the Superintendent of the Ratnagiri Lunatic Asylum, 3 March 1917, GD, 1917/82, MSA.

built at Naupada, Thana, replaced the Colaba asylum.[37] In 1913, the government opened the first central asylum of the Presidency at Yerawada, Poona.[38]

Colonial expectations regarding the asylum system were heterogeneous. The government envisioned a system that would confine dangerous, criminal, and wandering lunatics.[39] The penal and judicial departments saw asylums as an 'auxiliary to the penal system'.[40] The medical class wanted to establish an expansive medical system for mentally ill people.[41] Each agent in the colonial bureaucracy differed in their understanding of the function of the asylum as a colonial institution, leading to internal contestations between these agencies during its years of expansion. Power contestations ensured that superintendents in India never gained an 'all-embracing hegemony'.[42] The government assigned the task of the maintenance and management of asylums to the medical class who had to adhere to the two principles of 'cheapness and expediency'.[43] Superintendents played a crucial role in the asylum bureaucracy as they served as the chief link between patients, subordinate staff, and the government.

THE SUPERINTENDENT AND THE COLONIAL ASYLUM

The colonial government expected superintendents to perform three main functions: maintain surveillance and discipline, produce knowledge about Indian insanity,[44] and maintain a productive patient class. In executing

[37] From the Surgeon General to the Secretary of Government, 31 January 1902, GoB, GD, 1902/61, MSA.

[38] Triennial Report on the Lunatic Asylums in the Bombay Presidency, 1912–1914, p. 1, NLS.

[39] Waltraud Ernst, 'Out of Sight and Out of Mind: Insanity in Early 19th Century British India', in Joseph Melling and Bill Forsythe (eds.), *Insanity, Institutions and Society, 1800–1914: Studies in the Social History of Medicine* (London, New York: Routledge, 1991), p. 246.

[40] Foucault, *Power/Knowledge: Selected Interviews and Other Writings, 1972–1977*, p. 44.

[41] Waltraud Ernst, *Mad Tales from the Raj: Colonial Psychiatry in South Asia, 1800–58* (New York: Anthem Press, 2010), p. 53.

[42] Andrew Scull, 'Discovery of the Asylum Revisited: Lunacy Reform in the New American Republic', in Andrew Scull (ed.), *Madhouses, Mad-Doctors, and Madmen* (London: Athlone Press, 1981), p. 153.

[43] W.S. Jagoe Shaw, 'The Alienist Department of India', *British Journal of Psychiatry*, Vol. 78, April 1932, p. 334.

[44] James Mills, *Madness, Cannabis and Colonialism: The 'Native Only' Lunatic Asylums of British India, 1857–1900* (London: Macmillan Press Ltd., 2000), pp. 14, 65; Sanjeev Jain,

these functions, the superintendents ran into trouble with the government and its penal and judicial departments.

Surveillance and Discipline

Surveillance was crucial to the functioning of the colonial state. Surveillance facilitated the 'building of a body of knowledge' and enabled policing.[45] In the colonial context, this knowledge served to legitimize the British rule based on the 'self-validating' argument of Indian incapability for self-governance.[46] Surveillance facilitated the policing of deviant groups like 'sanyasis, sadhus, fakirs, dacoits, goondas, thugs, pastoralists, herders and entertainers'.[47] As colonial institutions, the government used lunatic asylums to execute surveillance for the purposes of gathering knowledge of Indian people and policing deviants. Foucault described asylums as institutions characterized by the 'spatial "nesting" of hierarchized surveillance'.[48]

Surveillance facilitated the creation of a body of knowledge about Indian people and patients.[49] As early as 1814, when Bombay's asylum system was in its nascent stages, the Medical Board asked Assistant Surgeon Maxwell, the newly appointed Superintendent of the Colaba Lunatic Asylum, to 'make out a report of the unfortunate people under ... [his] charge as soon as he had sufficient experience'.[50] Maxwell wrote detailed case notes stating his success in performing functions of surveillance and discipline through the observation of his patients. Month after month, he extensively reported the progress of patients under his surveillance and

'Psychiatry and Confinement in India', in Roy Porter and David Wright (eds.), *The Confinement of the Insane: International Perspectives, 1800–1965* (New York: Cambridge University Press, 2003), p. 283.

[45] Michel Foucault, *Discipline and Punish; the Birth of the Prison,* trans. Alan Sheridan (New York: Random House, 1977), pp. 171, 173, 294.

[46] Sanjay Nigam, 'Disciplining and Policing the "Criminals by Birth", Part 1: The Making of a Colonial Stereotype—The Criminal Tribes and Castes of North India', *The Indian Economic and Social History Review*, Vol. 27, No. 2, 1990, p. 133.

[47] Bernard Cohn, *Colonialism and its Forms of Knowledge: The British in India* (New Jersey: Princeton University Press, 1996), p. 10.

[48] Foucault, *Discipline and Punish,* p. 171.

[49] Foucault argued that 'there is no power relation without the correlative constitution of a field of knowledge, nor any knowledge that does not presuppose and constitute at the same time, power relations'. See Foucault, *Discipline and Punish,* p. 27.

[50] From Asst. Surgeon J.A. Maxwell to the Chief Secretary to the Government of Bombay, 4 June 1814, GoB, PDD, 1814/368, MSA.

treatment, which mainly entailed curing physical symptoms and reducing excitability in patients.[51] Even when the government established the new asylum in Ratnagiri in 1886, the Surgeon General emphasized that the observation of patients was crucial to its management.[52] Surveillance was a serious priority for the government that considered the duties of a superintendent as having 'more affinity with those of a superintendent of a prison than those of a Medical officer'.[53]

Superintendents worked in close conjunction with the subordinate asylum staff in performing surveillance duties. By the mid-nineteenth century, superintendents increasingly assigned surveillance tasks to their subordinate staff. In 1852, Superintendent Campbell recommended changes to the accommodation of staff within the asylum, since the distance between their accommodation and the asylum building meant that 'they were unable to exercise unremitting surveillance'. Dr. Campbell moved his staff to rooms closer to the patient wards so that they could hear them. He assigned a room to the European keeper that was closer to the galleries where he could keep vigilance over Indian staff and patients. Superintendent Campbell moved outside the asylum building to a bungalow at a distance (See Fig. 3.1). He justified his decision by stating that he was close enough to the eastern wing that housed those patients who needed 'the most constant and careful supervision' and they would still come under his 'immediate eye and ear'.[54]

Superintendents even engaged patients in the task of surveillance. In 1912, Jiva, a criminal patient at the Ratnagiri Asylum, murdered Babaji, a *cooly*[55] employed at the asylum. While sitting at his 'regular place' under the

---

[51] Dr. Maxwell records that blistering was extremely effective in treating patients whose symptoms included swelling. From Asst. Surgeon J.A. Maxwell to the Chief Secretary to the Government of Bombay, 4 June 1814, GoB, PDD, 1814/368, MSA.

[52] From the Surgeon General to the Secretary to the Government of Bombay, 26 February 1886, GoB, GD, 1886/58, MSA.

[53] Memorandum by the Commissioner of Sindh, No. 1819, 21 August 1895, Medical Proceedings, Government of India, Home Department, Simla Records, September 1897, Nos. 188–232, NAI.

[54] Report on the Lunatic Asylum at Colaba for the Year Ending 1852, GoB, GD, 1853/48, MSA.

[55] S.M. Edwardes describes the *cooly*. 'The *Naoghani* is a skilful workman, trained to deal with heavy loads and experienced in the manipulation of pulleys or blocks and always to be trusted for work that requires nerve. He is also known sometimes as a "bamboo-cooly"'. See S.M. Edwardes, *Gazetteer of Bombay City and Island*, Vol. 1 (Bombay: Times Press, 1909), p. 213; L. Dzuvichu described them as 'primitive tribes' who were employed in manual labour

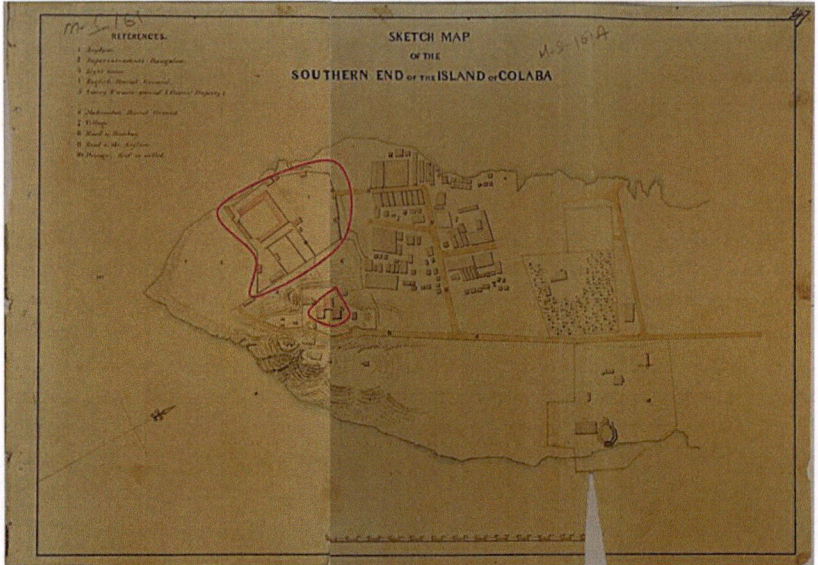

Fig. 3.1 The superintendent's new bungalow (2) located outside the walls of the Colaba Lunatic asylum (1). (Source: Report on the Lunatic Asylum at Colaba for the Year Ending 1852, GoB, GD, 1853/48, MSA)

watch of his warder, he suddenly began walking towards the workers who were fixing a water pipe. Jiva then picked a *pawrah*[56] and beat Babaji to death. The incident occurred while the superintendent was at the asylum. Superintendent A.G. Sargent defended himself before the Medical Board by stating that he gave the warders 'special orders to watch' Jiva.[57] He also collected the statements from the warder, other workers, and even two patients as evidence. Both patients in their statements recorded the beating and the fact that 'there was a peon close by'.[58] Based on the evidence that the superintendent, patients, and coolies presented, the Medical Board

for various public works in British India. See L. Dzuvichu, 'Empire on their Backs: Coolies in the Eastern Borderland of the British Raj', *IRSH*, Special Issue, Vol. 59, 2014, p. 91.

[56] *Pawrah*, also referred to as *pawada*, is an agricultural hoe used in farming and construction.

[57] From the Superintendent of the Ratnagiri Asylum to the Personal Asst. with the Government of Bombay, 15 August 1912, GoB, GD, 1912/95, MSA.

[58] Statement of Ganapaya Shankar, Patient, Ratnagiri Lunatic Asylum, 14 January 1912, GoB, GD, 1912/95, MSA; Statement of Shabas Shiwa Bhajwe, Patient, Ratnagiri Lunatic Asylum, 14 January 1912, GoB, GD, 1912/95, MSA.

ordered the warder Keshav's dismissal because he failed to act with 'ordinary courage and promptness'.[59] Superintendents used the 'native agency'[60] of subordinate staff and patients to exercise surveillance upon each other. Surveillance also facilitated the maintenance of discipline.

Bombay's superintendents maintained discipline through a system of rewards and punishments.[61] They punished or dismissed subordinate staff for their resistance to discipline or negligence. In a similar manner, they also rewarded staff when they maintained discipline and exercised surveillance. Punishments for patients included withdrawal of privileges like tobacco or amusements,[62] or even solitary confinement.[63] Dr. G. Bainbridge, Surgeon General with the Government of Bombay, explained:

> The unruly insanes are as much as possible induced to work by the knowledge that they will not otherwise be allowed to share in the diversions and other inducements provided.[64]

Asylum staff permitted or denied access to amusements based on patients' behaviour, which served as a disciplinary measure. Rewards also included small sums of money, tobacco, or extra food.[65] The Diet Chart for Bombay's Lunatic Asylums (Fig. 3.2) had provisions for rewarding patients who were willing to work with extra flour and bread.[66] While superintendents intended to use rewards and punishments to facilitate the employment of patients, they did not always succeed.

[59] From the Surgeon General with the Government of Bombay to the Secretary to Government of Bombay, 22 October 1912, GoB, GD, 1912/95, MSA.

[60] Lovett, 'The Development of the Services, 1858–1918', p. 362.

[61] Report on the Lunatic Asylum at Colaba for the Year Ending 1852, Government of Bombay, General Department, 1853/48, MSA, Mumbai. The Surgeon General records the practice of giving pocket money to patients for indulgences like tobacco. Patients were permitted to buy indulgences from the local bazar. Since the practice was 'highly prized by lunatics', the expenses were added to asylum's bills after the donation was withdrawn. From the Surgeon General, Indian Medical Department (IMD), to the Secretary to Government of Bombay, 23 February 1876, GoB, GD, 1876/55, MSA.

[62] Lyon Isidore Bernadotte, *Medical Jurisprudence for India, with Illustrative Cases*, Vol. 7 (Calcutta: Thacker and Spink, 1921), p. 363.

[63] Extract from the Daily Register of Solitary [Confinement], Ratnagiri Lunatic Asylum, 1912, GoB, GD, 1912/95, MSA.

[64] APR, 1899, p. 12, NLS.

[65] Native Diet Scale of the Bombay Lunatic Asylums, attached to the Rules of the Bombay Lunatic Asylum, 1864, GoB, GD,1862–1864/15, MSA.

[66] Rules of the Bombay Lunatic Asylum, 1864, GoB, GD, 1862–1864/15, MSA.

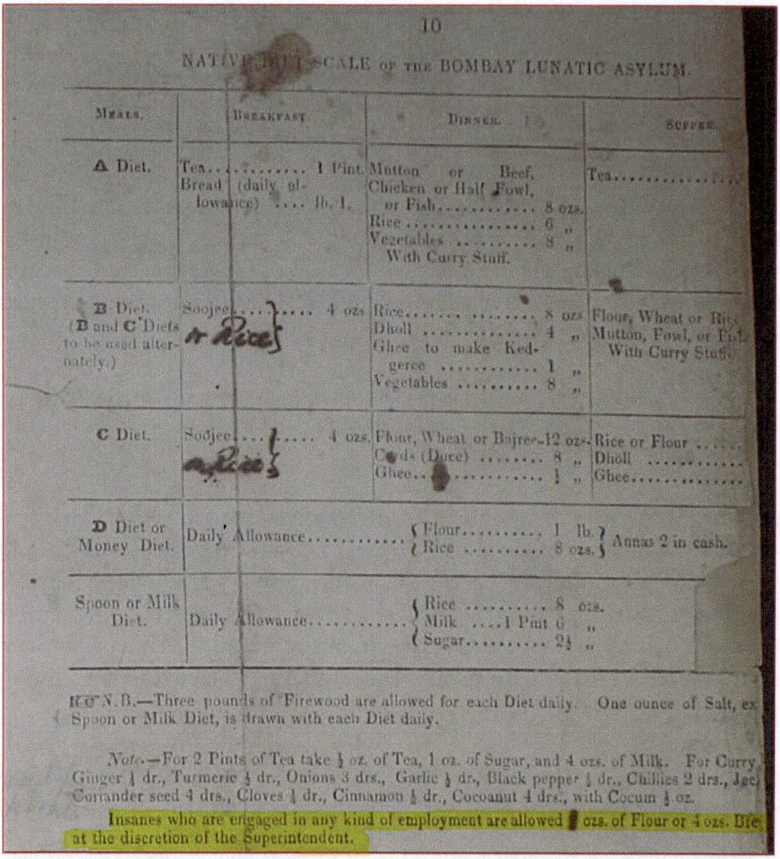

10

NATIVE DIET SCALE OF THE BOMBAY LUNATIC ASYLUM.

MEALS.	BREAKFAST.	DINNER.	SUPPER.
A Diet.	Tea............ 1 Pint. Bread (daily allowance) .... lb. 1.	Mutton or Beef, Chicken or Half Fowl, or Fish............ 8 ozs. Rice .... 6 ,, Vegetables .... 8 ,, With Curry Stuff.	Tea................
B Diet. (B and C Diets to be used alternately.)	Soojee...... 4 ozs. or Rice	Rice................ 8 ozs. Dholl .... 4 ,, Ghee to make Kedgeree .... 1 ,, Vegetables .... 8 ,,	Flour, Wheat or Ri[illegible] Mutton, Fowl, or Fi[illegible] With Curry Stuff.
C Diet.	Soojee...... 4 ozs. or Rice	Flour, Wheat or Bajree–12 ozs. Curds (Duee) .... 8 ,, Ghee.............. 1 ,,	Rice or Flour ...... Dholl .... Ghee............
D Diet or Money Diet.	Daily Allowance............	Flour.......... 1 lb. Rice .... 8 ozs.	Annas 2 in cash.
Spoon or Milk Diet.	Daily Allowance............	Rice .... 8 ozs. Milk ....1 Pint 6 ,, Sugar.......... 2½ ,,	

N.B.—Three pounds of Firewood are allowed for each Diet daily. One ounce of Salt, ex[illegible] Spoon or Milk Diet, is drawn with each Diet daily.

Note.—For 2 Pints of Tea take ½ oz. of Tea, 1 oz. of Sugar, and 4 ozs. of Milk. For Curry, Ginger ¼ dr., Turmeric ½ dr., Onions 3 drs., Garlic ½ dr., Black pepper ¼ dr., Chillies 2 drs., Jee[illegible] Corriander seed 4 drs., Cloves ¼ dr., Cinnamon ¼ dr., Cocoanut 4 drs., with Cocum ½ oz.

Insanes who are engaged in any kind of employment are allowed [illegible] ozs. of Flour or 4 ozs. Bre[illegible] at the discretion of the Superintendent.

Fig. 3.2 Native Diet Scale for the asylums in the Bombay Presidency showing extra quantities of food permitted to those patients who maintained discipline through occupation. (Source: Rules of the Bombay Lunatic Asylum, 1864, GoB, GD, 1862–1864/15, MSA)

Bombay's superintendents often found the task of maintaining surveillance and discipline challenging. Major Campbell, Superintendent at Colaba, reported three cases of escape between 1849 and 1853; he blamed them on the lack of boundary walls around the asylum and the negligence of staff.[67] At the close of the nineteenth century, Surgeon

[67] From Superintendent, Colaba Lunatic Asylum, to the Secretary, Medical Board, 26 October 1853, GoB, GD, 1853/48, MSA.

James Cleghorn, Director General of the IMS, expressed dismay at the absence of 'method and discipline in the arrangements connected with the engagement of the inmates and the uproar and confusion present that was in contrast to the quietness and order of a well-managed asylum'.[68]

Superintendents had little motivation to maintain a panopticon[69] version of surveillance and discipline within asylum walls. Asylum superintendence was not an esteemed job and superintendents considered it as one of the minor 'prizes of the service',[70] especially because of petty salaries superintendents received.[71] *Gharry* allowances or visiting charges paid to superintendents often permitted only limited visits to the asylum. Additional expenses paid to superintendents often only covered travelling costs to the asylum.[72] Besides, asylum superintendence came under the 'additional charge' of the civil surgeon.[73] Secretary of State for India Mr. John Morley tried to change the convention, but the system continued due to 'financial stress'.[74] Furthermore, superintendents were highly dependent on the untrained subordinate staff who they employed because it was difficult to get 'attendants from a good class'. Even overseers were 'elderly men with their best energies gone' and forced to work out of necessity.[75] The laxity in surveillance also affected knowledge production in the asylum.

---

[68] Note by the Director General, IMS, on the reports of Lunatic Asylums, under Local Governments and Administrations for the Year 1895, Medical Proceedings, Government of India, Home Department, Simla Records, September 1896, Nos. 65–90, NAI.

[69] Bentham's panopticon style envisioned buildings designed specially to execute constant surveillance over those detained. See John Bowring (ed.), *The Works of Jeremy Bentham*, Vol. 4. (Edinburgh: William Tait, 1843), pp. 65, 69; Foucault, *Discipline and Punish: The Birth of the Prison*, p. 200.

[70] Report on the Lunatic Asylum at Colaba for the Year Ending 1852, GoB, GD, 1853/48, MSA.

[71] From Lt. Col. Barry, Superintendent, Colaba Lunatic Asylum, to the Personal Asst. to the Surgeon General with the Government of Bombay, 25 June 1904, GoB, GD, 1907/81, MSA.

[72] From Lt. Col. Barry, Superintendent, Colaba Lunatic Asylum, to the Personal Asst. to the Surgeon General with the Government of Bombay, 25 June 1904, GoB, GD, 1907/81, MSA.

[73] Shaw, 'The Alienist Department', p. 336.

[74] Ibid., p. 335.

[75] From Lt. Col. Barry, Superintendent, Colaba Lunatic Asylum, to the Personal Asst. to the Surgeon General with the Government of Bombay, 25 June 1904, GoB, GD, 1907/81, MSA.

Production of Knowledge

The *Indian Medical Gazette* described India as a lucrative site for knowledge production. It elaborated:

> That India forms a fruitful field of medico-legal observations is somewhat a trite saying to those who know the country and is obviously proved by the rich storehouse of facts accumulated in the numerous series of reports, papers and textbooks dealing with medical jurisprudence.[76]

Knowledge was necessary for maintaining and justifying colonial rule in India, and the government used colonial asylums as centres for knowledge production.[77] For asylums to work as a colonial disciplinary system, it was necessary for power and knowledge to work in a circular process 'reinforcing' each other. Knowledge produced from these asylums served as common knowledge about Indian people, and the government used it in governing the colony. For example, as James Mills argued, the government considered the knowledge produced by observing patients who suffered from insanity as descriptive of hemp users all over India.[78] The colonial state expected superintendents to 'create knowledge' through their observation of Indian patients which would be used to 'reinforce'[79] colonial power. Thus colonial power facilitated knowledge production and knowledge served to justify the need for a benevolent colonial rule.

Lunatic asylums were important sites of producing knowledge that was essential for understanding the Indian populace. Superintendents were often 'pressed to give statistical information'.[80] The type of knowledge that the colonial state sought was a description of mental illness in Indians that would strengthen strongly held colonial prejudices towards Indians. Few superintendents produced comparative studies between western and

---

[76] W.J. Buchanan (ed.), *The Indian Medical Gazette. A Monthly Journal of Medicine, Surgery, Public Health, and General Medical Intelligence, Indian and European*, Vol. XXXIX (Calcutta: Spink and Co., 1904), p. 113.

[77] James Mills, *Madness, Cannabis and Colonialism: The 'Native Only' Lunatic Asylums of British India, 1857–1900* (London: Macmillan Press Ltd., 2000), pp. 14, 65.

[78] Foucault, *Discipline and Punish*, p. 224.

[79] Ibid.

[80] The Hemp Commission Report elaborated that superintendents '[had] been so pressed to give statistical information that they have done so without considering whether it could[was] be scientific'. See Report of the Indian Hemp Drugs Commission, 1894–1895, Vol. 1, p. 236, NLS.

Indian insanity. Major Overbeck-Wright, Superintendent of the Agra Asylum, made comparisons on the state of insanity in India and Britain and concluded: 'Insanity in India is at least as rife as in Britain'.[81] The emphasis of these comparative studies was on proving the high prevalence of insanity in India.

In colonial India throughout the nineteenth century, the British endeavoured to systematically record and classify the Indian population.[82] The systematic recording and classification of asylum patients started as early as 1814. Dr. Maxwell, in his case notes, provides monthly description on the progress and health of his patients.[83] By the mid-nineteenth century, an increased recording of patients occurs. Dr. Campbell wrote detailed letters to the government reporting the condition of the asylum and his patients.[84] Superintendents not only maintained case notes and patient registers but also wrote Annual Reports to the government. From the 1870s, asylum agencies maintained more elaborate Annual Asylum Reports. Colonial agencies typed these reports, unlike the handwritten letter reports of the previous decades. These reports contained information about the financial and physical condition of the asylum and its treatment practices. The reports also contained tables that classified patients based on race, sex, occupation, and religion.[85] Reports were a common way for the British to collect information on colonial subjects.

By 1902, the government sent the information gathered in colonial asylums to asylums in Britain for producing comparative studies on western and Indian insanity. Clive Bradley, a Medical Officer at the Colney Hatch, London County Lunatic Asylum, wrote to the Governor of Bombay:

> Collecting information as I am in all parts of the world concerning the mentally afflicted(insane), I should be deeply obliged if you could kindly have me informed of the following points, as regards to the Province of Bombay.

[81] A.W. Overbeck Wright, *Mental Derangements in India: Its Symptoms and Treatment* (Calcutta and Simla: Thacker, Spink and Co., 1912), pp. 98–103.

[82] Cohn, *Colonialism and its Forms of Knowledge*, p. 11.

[83] From Asst. Surgeon J.A. Maxwell to the Chief Secretary to the Government of Bombay, 4 June 1814, GoB, PDD, 1814/368, MSA.

[84] Report on the Lunatic Asylum at Colaba for the Year Ending 1852, GoB, GD, 1853/48, MSA.

[85] See APR 1873–1900, NLS.

1. What is the number of special institutions or the insane.
2. What is the **number of insane persons of each race**, who are at present confined in Bombay or in other institutions.
3. What is the **number or portions of the insanes of different races**
4. To what extent does insanity prevail among the general population of the Province, not in confinement.
5. What are the **principal forms of mental disease among the natives.**
6. What are the chief causes assigned for mental disease.[86]

In response to Officer Bradley's letter, the Governor sent him the Annual Asylum Progress Reports as a conclusive source for his investigations on Indian insanity.[87] Such comparative studies based on asylum records showed a very small number of admissions in Indian asylums compared to their British counterparts.

Low asylum admissions left both doctors and the state baffled. The prevalence of high rates of mental illness among Indian communities, if proven through asylum records, would justify the need for a benevolent colonial rule. Nevertheless, asylum records proved otherwise. The colonial state therefore attributed low numbers of Indian patients in asylums to Indians possessing 'less brain energy' and to the 'lower state of civilization'.[88] Colonial observers also attributed poor admissions to the fact that Indians did not know how to recognize insanity, since they did not consider deaf mutes or religious mendicants insane.[89] While the government tried to gather information from asylums, the process of the production of knowledge through asylums often faced disruptions.

Superintendents faced several obstacles while studying Indian insanity. Superintendents themselves used asylum records to learn first-hand the treatment and management of their patients. However, constant transfers meant that superintendents were unable to apply the knowledge acquired

---

[86] From Clive Bradley, Medical Officer, Colney Hatch, London County Lunatic Asylum, to the Governor of Bombay, 17 October 1902, GD, 1902/54, MSA. Text highlighted for emphasis.

[87] From the Secretary to the Government of Bombay to Clive Bradley, Medical Officer, Colney Hatch, London County Lunatic Asylum, 7 November 1902, GoB, GD, 1902/54, MSA.

[88] From Curzon of Kedleston, E.H. Collen, A.C. Trevor, C.M. Rivaz, E.F. Law to the Secretary of State for India, Simla, 19 July 1900, Government of India, Finance and Commerce Department, GoB, GD, 1901/66, MSA.

[89] Bernadotte, *Medical Jurisprudence for India*, pp. 353–354.

by them to reform treatment methods.[90] Furthermore, the government did not give them any incentives to pursue the study of insanity. It did not consider the production of knowledge and even professional capabilities as criteria for remuneration. Superintendent Barry complained of the inconsistency in salaries of superintendents. A layman appointed as deputy superintendent at the Bhawanipur asylum in Bengal received Rs. 250 a month, while Superintendent Barry with his 'double University qualification' and experience was paid Rs. 100. Superintendent Barry's assistant surgeon received a salary of Rs. 180.[91] Apart from these factors, the medical class noted in 1852 that larger groups of patients were needed to study insanity better. The Medical Board therefore proposed the building of larger asylums that would provide access to larger groups of mentally ill people.[92] The medical class made constant petitions to the government for the expansion of the asylum system. The expansion would facilitate the observation of a larger number of patients to produce knowledge.[93] The government heeded the petition of the medical class for a large asylum only in 1913, when it established the first central asylum in Yerawada, Poona.[94]

The failure on the part of the superintendents to produce enough knowledge about categories of Indian insanity created a power contest among colonial agents who clashed with each other to claim expert knowledge on Indian insanity. In 1849, Magistrate Bettington sent a Brahmin, Devram, to the asylum in Ahmedabad, since he refused to eat for certain days as a mode of ritual fasting. Magistrate Bettington concluded that his fast was an attempt at suicide.[95] Assistant Surgeon Gillanders, who was responsible for the insane hospital at Ahmedabad, after observing him, was convinced of the Brahmin's sanity. Surgeon Gillanders pleaded for his

[90] Report on the Lunatic Asylum at Colaba for the Year Ending 1852, GoB, GD, 1853/48, MSA.

[91] From Lt. Col. Barry, Superintendent, Colaba Lunatic Asylum, to the Personal Asst. to the Surgeon General with the Government of Bombay, 25 June 1904, GoB, GD, 1907/81, MSA.

[92] From the Secretary of Medical Board to the Commissioner of Scind, 3 June 1851, GoB, GD, 1852/10, MSA.

[93] Surgeon General with the Government of Bombay to Secretary to the Government of Bombay, 26 February 1886, GoB, GD, 1886/58, MSA.

[94] Triennial Report on the Lunatic Asylums in the Bombay Presidency, 1912–1914, p. 1, NLS.

[95] From the Magistrate of Ahmedabad to the Superintending Surgeon, Ahmedabad, 15 August 1849, JD, GoB, GD, 1849/38, MSA.

release, since Devram's brother was willing to care for him.[96] However, for several months, Brahmin Devram remained in the asylum, as the duel between Magistrate Bettington and the Assistant Surgeon continued.[97] Because the penal and judicial departments perceived the asylum as an 'auxiliary to the penal system',[98] they contested the agency of the medical class. Disagreements between magistrates, commissioners of police, and superintendents continued right through the nineteenth and early twentieth centuries. Judicial and penal agencies were most often the first link between the patients and the colonial asylum, and they contested the authority of superintendents regarding the knowledge of mental illness. The government authorized them to define the symptoms of a person's mental illness or act as witnesses to their insanity. In several instances, the Hemp Commission noted that while a medical officer issued a lunacy certificate, the descriptive role was filled out by a police officer, even by a *chowkidar* (watchman) or *havildar* (police constable).[99]

The government tactfully handled the power contestation between the penal departments and the medical class. The government on several occasions mediated between magistrates, police, and the superintendents. For example, overcrowding created a need for expansion of the asylum system that was not economical to undertake. In 1851, a government circular dissuaded magistrates from the 'indiscriminate admission of patients'.[100] Magistrates objected to the circular, stating that it was 'incompatible with the purpose' for which the asylum was founded and was 'destructive to its utility'.[101] Since the state prioritized economical spending of the state budget over the care of people suffering from mental illness, they supported superintendents in their decision to turn away patients sent by magistrates. The state also occasionally imposed collaboration between asylum superintendents and the judicial and penal departments. The Hemp Commission was one such experiment in collaboration. The government made superintendents collaborate with experienced magistrates in making inquiries

[96] From Asst. Surgeon Gillanders to the Superintending Surgeon, Ahmedabad, 22 January 1850, GoB, GD, 1849/38, MSA.

[97] From the Bombay Medical Board Office to the Secretary to the Government of Bombay, GoB, GD, 1849/38, MSA.

[98] Foucault, *Power/Knowledge: Selected Interviews and Other Writings, 1972–1977*, p. 4.

[99] Report of the Indian Hemp Drugs Commission, 1894–1895, Vol. 1, p. 23, NLS.

[100] Circular to All Magistrates, 22 November 1851, GoB, GD, 1851/15, MSA.

[101] Senior Magistrate of Police, Bombay, to the Secretary to the Government, 3 July 1849, Government of Bombay, Board's Collection, 1851–1852, F4/2450, IOR, BL, London.

into personal case histories to determine links between hemp and insani-ty.[102] The contention between the superintendents and the penal and judi-cial departments continued into the twentieth century. In 1917, the government passed another resolution that notified magistrates to inform superintendents in advance before the courts or the police sent anyone to a government asylum.[103]

The colonial state also contested the agency of the superintendents, as it challenged their knowledge as medical professionals. Superintendents often 'failed to convince government and medical authorities of their spe-cial professional skills'.[104] While they produced more organized and detailed reports after 1870, the government concluded that the reports were based on statistics that were not 'trustworthy'.[105] Hemp commis-sioners criticized superintendents for regarding 'statistics as merely clerical work of no practical importance'[106] and for producing unreliable statistics and submitting them 'year after year in asylum reports'.[107] In 1895, the Hemp Commission noted: 'Entries would be laughable but for a fact they indicate[d] a lamentable absence of anything like the systematic treatment of mental disease by superintendents'.[108] It also vilified superintendents for not having 'knowledge about the links between hemp and insanity'.[109] Moreover, the Director General of the IMS stated that the classification of different types of insanity in the reports was 'rather confusing'.[110] The

---

[102] Report of the Indian Hemp Drugs Commission, 1894–1895, Vol. 1, p. 7, NLS.

[103] Government Resolution, Bombay Castle, 6 June 1917, GoB, GD, 1917/773, MSA.

[104] Waltraud Ernst made this argument for the first half of the nineteenth century. See Waltraud Ernst, *Mad Tales from the Raj*, p. 86. However, even at the close of the century the Hemp Commission noted that asylum superintendents had made little progress compared to their counterparts in England. The superintendents failed to make a 'special study of insan-ity'. From the Government of Bengal to the Home Department, Government of India, Administration of Lunatic Asylums in India, 25 August 1896, Medical Proceedings–August, Simla Records 4, Home Department, 1897, Nos. 188–232, NAI.

[105] Report of the Indian Hemp Drugs Commission, 1894–1895, Vol. 1, p. 227, NLS.

[106] A.H.L. Fraser and C.J.H. Warden, Notes on Asylum Administration, 7 August 1894, GoB, GD, 1895/77, MSA.

[107] Report of the Indian Hemp Drugs Commission, 1894–1895, Vol. 1, p. 230, NLS.

[108] A.H.L. Fraser and C.J.H. Warden, Notes on Asylum Administration, 7 August 1894, GoB, GD, 1895/77, MSA.

[109] A.H.L. Fraser and C.J.H. Warden, Notes on Asylum Administration, 7 August 1894, GoB, GD, 1895/77, MSA.

[110] Note by the Director General, IMS, on the Reports of Lunatic Asylums under Local Governments and Administrations for the year 1895, Medical Proceedings, Government of India, Home Department, Simla Records, September 1896, Nos. 65–90, NAI.

inefficiency of superintendents meant that asylum statistics were unreliable and several gaps existed in the knowledge of mental illness among Indians. The colonial state attempted to fill in the gaps in the knowledge of Indian insanity created by the failure of asylum superintendents, for the 'expansion of knowledge was not so much a by-product of the empire as a condition for it'.[111] The colonial state set up the Hemp Commission with the intent of establishing a new type of insanity specific to Indian people. The commission elaborately studied links between Indian hemp and 'native insanity'. The outcome of the Hemp Commission Report was a 'collection of a body of information about these selected cases far superior to anything heretofore available'.[112] However, Bombay's medical authorities staunchly defended their superintendents despite the scathing criticism from the Hemp commissioners. One surgeon noted that since 'no lunacy expert sat on the commission', the findings were not conclusive.[113] The Surgeon General of Bombay argued that the Hemp Commission Report was an 'exaggeration by officers with no experience of asylums in India'.[114] Constant government surveillance and interference in the agency of superintendents left them disgruntled. The government challenged the agency of the superintendents within the bureaucracy, instead of 'renewing and reaffirming' the 'power relations' between them.[115]

Maintaining a Productive Patient Class

The colonial state expected superintendents to maintain a productive patient class. Employing patients in manual work would ensure the inexpensive expansion and maintenance of asylums. Superintendents increasingly emphasized moral therapy over the nineteenth century. Occupation was the chief means of moral therapy and they used it conveniently to.

---

[111] C.A. Bayly, *Empire and Information: Intelligence Gathering and Social Communication in India, 1780–1870* (New York: Cambridge University Press, 1996), p. 56.

[112] Report of the Indian Hemp Drugs Commission, 1894–1895, Vol. 1, p. 238, NLS.

[113] John Warnock, 'Insanity from Hasheesh', *British Journal of Psychiatry*, Vol. 49, January 1903, p. 96.

[114] From the Surgeon General with the Government of Bombay, 18 July 1895, Simla, Records 4, Home Department, Medical Proceedings, August 1897, Nos. 188–232, NAI.

[115] 'Power is seen as a more volatile, unstable element, which can be always contested, so power relations must be permanently renewed and reaffirmed.' See Sergiu Balan, 'Foucault's View on Power Relations', *Cogito: Multidisciplinary Research Journal*, Vol. 2, No. 2, June 2010, p. 42.

justify the employment of patients on the pretext of therapy. Occupation included 'household duties, scrubbing and cleaning the rooms and galleries, sweeping the ground, gardening, the different branches of *Ratlan* (wicker or cane) work, mat making, rope spinning, weaving, rope making, straw plaiting'.[116] Patients were also employed in cane work, carpentry, and tailoring. Women were engaged in '[c]orn grinding and needle work'.[117] Labouring patients helped maintain and expand the asylum system.

While trying to maintain a productive patient class, superintendents often found their authority challenged by local communities and even by patients. Superintendents blamed caste prejudices as an obstacle to getting patients engaged in work within the asylum.[118] It was a common practice at the Colaba Asylum to make patients carry provisions from commissariat stores because it amounted 'to the domestic value of 7 servants'.[119] However, in 1871, the *Akbari Sowdagar,* a vernacular newspaper, objected to the practice of patients being used to carry provisions from the commissariat stores during the 'sultry hours' of the day.[120] The government showed no empathy towards the challenges faced by superintendents. Instead, it blamed the lack of 'discipline and method' within the asylum on the inability of superintendents to find suitable 'employment and amusement' for the patients.[121]

Constant power contestations between the government, its judicial and penal departments, and the medical class led to a fragmented asylum bureaucracy. The inability of superintendents to exert surveillance, maintain discipline, produce knowledge, and maintain a productive patient class affected their position within the colonial hierarchy. The government was reserved in its support of superintendents because they had failed to fulfil its expectations. Superintendents themselves came under strict surveillance, combined with criticism and meagre funding for asylums. The

---

[116]Report on the Lunatic Asylum at Colaba for the Year Ending 1852, GoB, GD, 1853/48, MSA; APR, 1873–1874, p. 17, NLS.

[117]APR, 1878, p. 7, NLS.

[118]From the Asst. Surgeon, Lunatic Asylum Colaba, to the Medical Board, 21 February 1847, GoB, GD, 1847/41, MSA.

[119]APR, 1873–1874, p. 6, NLS.

[120]RNP, *Akbari Sowdagar*, 13 April 1871, K 406, J–D, PG 1–543, GoB, MSA.

[121]Note by the Director General, IMS, on the Reports of Lunatic Asylums under Local Governments and Administrations for the Year 1895, Medical Proceedings, Government of India, Home Department, Simla Records, September 1896, Nos. 65–90, NAI.

lack of support meant that the superintendents began displaying an increasing sense of disconnectedness towards the colonial state and an increasing connectedness towards Indians in Bombay's asylums, facilitating the creation of the 'middle ground'.[122]

EVOLUTION OF THE COLONIAL ASYLUM AS 'MIDDLE GROUND'[123]

In every human interaction, power is subject to negotiation ...[124]

Richard White argued that as the Algonquian and the French 'worlds' met, their interaction led to the development of a 'common ground or middle ground' between them. The middle ground developed as the French gained real knowledge about the Algonquians compared to their European counterparts who had the image of the Indians as 'savages'. The French and the Algonquians each failed to gain hegemony over the other; however, they continued in their relations since both groups needed each other to meet 'specific ends',[125] leading to the creation of a space of 'common conventions' also called the 'middle ground'. The middle ground led to a set of 'mutual inventions' which were justified in terms of what they perceived to be 'their partner's cultural premise'.[126] Using the concept of the 'middle ground', this section argues that within the colony, the asylum institution functioned as a 'middle ground' between colonial and local agencies. While political hegemony was achieved over India, the asylum represented a negotiated space rather than a hegemonized one.

Bombay, for Europeans in the nineteenth century, represented a socio-political and cultural middle ground. William Hunter, in his book on the history of Bombay's administration, stated:

> The competition of races, European and Indian ... is tempered by common interests, mutual forbearance and [in] certain reciprocal respect[s] imparts a moderation to Bombay's public opinion.[127]

---

[122] White, *The Middle Ground*.

[123] Ibid.

[124] Balan, 'Foucault's View on Power Relations', p. 61.

[125] See White, *The Middle Ground*, p. 51.

[126] While the French and Algonquians never achieved hegemony over each other, the British achieved politically hegemony over India. See White, *The Middle Ground*, pp. 51–53.

[127] Wilson, *Bombay 1885 to 1890*, p. 14.

Attitudes of 'mutual forbearance' and 'certain reciprocal respects' were also reflected in 'everyday'[128] asylum relations.[129] As Indian and colonial 'worlds' collided within asylum walls, superintendents increasingly compromised with the 'colonial' agenda of running a disciplinary system in order to civilize[130] and colonize 'native body and mind'.[131] In their experience with the Indian patients, superintendents concluded that they 'had to arrive at a common conception of suitable ways of acting'[132] in the colonial asylum. The 'middle ground' was a result of the adoption of local customs and practices within asylum walls. For superintendents, the creation of the 'middle ground' was a realistic scheme to ensure the survival of the asylum system and make its use more appealing to local communities. While holding strongly to their colonial self-understanding and racial superiority, they also showed an increasing connectedness to local practices, customs, and people, permitting their free expressions and even endorsing them as effective in the treatment process. The creation of this 'middle ground' left the colonial state disgruntled, since it interfered with the maintenance of a colonial disciplinary system. The asylum as a 'middle ground' represented a disjuncture between the colonial state and asylum superintendents. In some colonial asylums, like the Ranchi Indian Mental Hospital, western-educated Indian doctors ultimately hegemonized the asylum 'middle ground' in the later decades of the twentieth century. However, Bombay's asylums did not transform into colonial 'bastions'[133] in the early twentieth century.

The characteristics of the middle ground were evident in the relations between asylum superintendents and their subordinate staff. The mutual reliance between them served both groups 'to achieve quite specific ends'.[134] Superintendents supported their subordinate staff in their

---

[128]White, *The Middle Ground*, p. 55.

[129]Wilson, *Bombay 1885 to 1890*, p. 15.

[130]James Mills, '"More Important to Civilise than Subdue"? Lunatic Asylums, Psychiatric Practice and Fantasies of the "Civilising Mission" in British India 1858—1900', in Harald Fischer-Tiné and Michael Mann (eds.), *Colonialism as Civilising Mission* (London: Anthem Press, 2003), p. 190.

[131]Waltraud Ernst, 'Medical/Colonial Power-Lunatic Asylum in Bengal, c.1800–1900', *Journal of Asian History*, Vol. 40, No. 1, 2006, p. 79.

[132]White, *The Middle Ground*, p. 50.

[133]Anouska Bhattacharyya, 'Indian Insanes, Lunacy in the "Native" Asylums of Colonial India, 1858–1912', PhD Thesis, Harvard University, 2013, p. 211.

[134]White, *The Middle Ground*, p. 51.

demands for an increase in pay.[135] Superintendents even lobbied for better facilities for recreation and travel benefits like railway passes for their
subordinate staff.[136] While they prioritized European staff and gave them
more benefits, superintendents expressed a general concern for all their
subordinate staff. Superintendent Barry lamented that the isolation of
the Thana Asylum and the climate were detrimental to the health of his
subordinate staff. The isolated location of asylum meant that the 'native
servants' could not even have a 'few hours of fun'.[137] Four of his subordinate staff including a 'stalwart *ayah*' (a female clerk/wardress mostly
employed for menial work in the asylum) died after the asylum was moved
from Colaba to Naupada,[138] and his Assistant Surgeon, he added, had
drifted into a 'brooding melancholy'. Superintendents expounded that
the work of warders was 'arduous as they have often to work day and
night'.[139] At Colaba, explained Superintendent Barry, 'we are slave driv-
ing our establishment and this cannot be good for the mad'.[140] While
superintendents staunchly defended their subordinate staff, they also distanced themselves from them when they were negligent or inefficient.
Despite their negligence and 'alcoholic infirmities', the subordinate staff
were tolerated, since it was extremely difficult to find local people to staff
asylums.[141]

---

[135] Lt. Col. W.G.H. Henderson petitioning for an increase in pay for his staff explained: 'To
induce them to remain, emoluments must be raised'. From Lt. Col. W.G.H. Henderson,
IMS, Superintendent, Lunatic Asylum, Poona, to the Personal Asst. of the Surgeon General
with the Government of Bombay, 18 July, 1904, GoB, GD, 1907/81, MSA.

[136] Subordinate staff recruited from outside Sindh were granted free railway passes. From
the Secretary to Government of Bombay, General Department to the Secretary to the
Government of India, 23 November 1920, Home Department, Government of India,
Medical Proceedings, December 1920, Nos. 55–56, NAI; From Lt. Col. Barry,
Superintendent, Colaba Lunatic Asylum, to the Personal Asst. to the Surgeon General with
the Government of Bombay, 25 June 1904, GoB, GD, 1907/81, MSA.

[137] From Lt. Col. J.P. Barry, Superintendent, Colaba Lunatic Asylum, to the Personal Asst.
to the Surgeon General with the Government of Bombay, 25 June 1904, GoB, GD,
1907/81, MSA.

[138] Indian patients and staff were moved to the new 'native' asylum at Thana.

[139] From the Superintendent, Lunatic Asylum, Ahmedabad, to the Personal Asst. to the
Surgeon General Government of Bombay, 11 August 1912, GoB, GD, 1913/99, MSA.

[140] From Lt. Col. J. P. Barry, Superintendent, Colaba Lunatic Asylum, for the information
of the Official Visitors, 20 May 1904, GoB, GD, 1904/57, MSA.

[141] From Lt. Col. J.P. Barry, Superintendent, Colaba Lunatic Asylum, to the Personal Asst.
to the Surgeon General with the Government of Bombay, 25 June 1904, GoB, GD,
1907/81, MSA.

Subordinate staff continued to work in asylums for monetary gain and ascent in social status. Most of the subordinate staff in Bombay's asylums came from the *Mahar* and *Madrasi*[142] communities.[143] Indian society considered the Mahars 'dalit' or 'untouchable' during colonial times; they were a community who 'ran errands for the villages'.[144] While pay, promotions, and accommodation were good incentives for the subordinate staff, service in the asylum gave them a means to break free from 'economic and psychological subservience to existing village structures'.[145] Employment in the 'colonial apparatus'[146] provided them with an opportunity to repudiate the 'stranglehold of caste'.[147] Their service in colonial institutions also raised their status in the colonial social hierarchy. Colonial observers called them 'warm friends of the British government' who were 'not to be pitted by us against other classes of society, but to be upheld in their just rights and privileges'.[148] Historians have traditionally placed the responsibility of colonial domination of India on the British and the Indian bourgeoisie.[149] Loyalty to the British government, however, superseded class lines. In the case of the lunatic asylum, the staff came from the lower classes and castes who acted as colonial agents. Since their agency was indispensable to the functioning of the colonial asylum system, superintendents were willing to negotiate with them. Superintendents did not restrict their negotiations merely to Indian staff. They permitted some negotiations with patients and their relatives as well (Fig. 3.3).

Over the nineteenth century, superintendents displayed an increasing connectedness towards Indian patients and their families, 'mutually inventing' new conventions in Bombay's asylums. Within the colonial asylum, superintendents were accommodating towards local social customs.

---

[142] The Mahars were a community from Maharashtra, they were traditionally considered as untouchable and any local from Madras is referred to as a Madrasi.

[143] From Lt. Col. Barry, Superintendent, Colaba Lunatic Asylum, to the Personal Asst. to the Surgeon General with the Government of Bombay, 25 June 1904, GoB, GD, 1907/81, MSA.

[144] M.T. Joseph, SVD, 'Migration and Identity formation: A Case study of Dalit Assertion in Aurangabad, Maharashtra', in Jose Joseph and L. Stanislaus (eds.), *Migration and Mission in India* (New Delhi: ISPCK, 2007), p. 101.

[145] Joseph, 'Migration and Identity formation', p. 103.

[146] Ibid., p. 102.

[147] Ibid., p. 104.

[148] William Johnson, *The Oriental Races and Tribes, Residents and Visitors of Bombay: A Series of Photographs with Letter-press Descriptions*, Vol. 2 (London: W.J. Johnson, 1866), p. 67.

[149] Ranajit Guha, *Dominance Without Hegemony: History and Power in Colonial India* (Cambridge, London: Harvard University Press, 1997), p. 100.

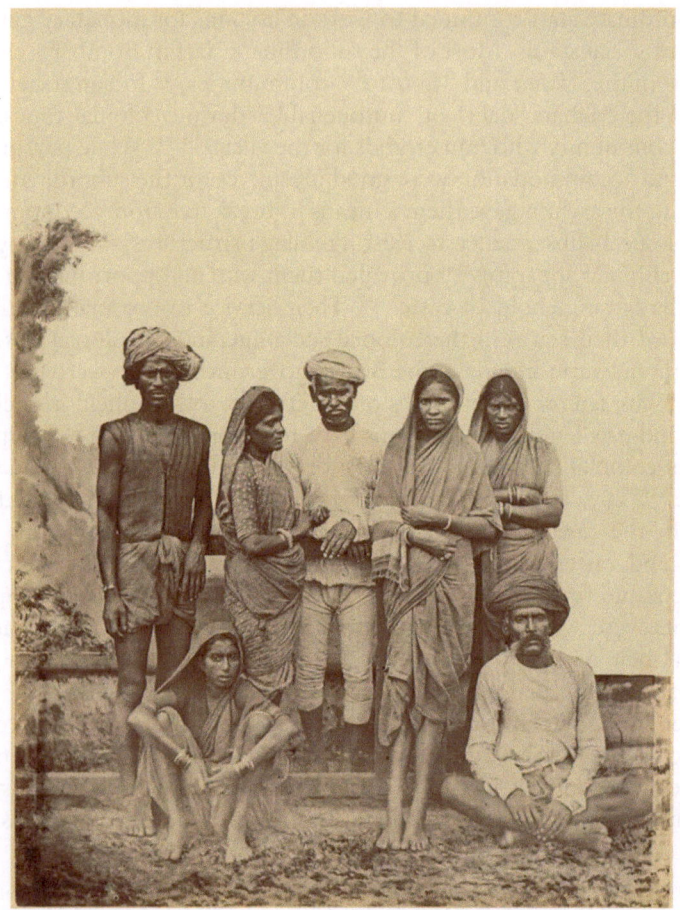

Fig. 3.3 The Mahar community that formed most of the subordinate staff in Bombay's asylums. (Source: William Johnson, *The Oriental Races and Tribes, Residents and Visitors of Bombay: A Series of Photographs with Letter-press Descriptions*, Vol. 2 (London: W.J. Johnson, 1866), p. 6)

Superintendent Campbell reported that patients at the Colaba Asylum were permitted to cook at an hour and in a manner 'that was agreeable to their feelings'.[150] He gave patients an allowance to buy food if they refused

---

[150] Report on the Lunatic Asylum at Colaba for the Year Ending 1852, GoB, GD, 1853/48, MSA, Mumbai; From the Superintendent, Lunatic Asylum, Colaba, to the Secretary to the Principal Inspector General, Medical Department, 31 July 1863, GoB, GD, 1862–1864/15, MSA.

their asylum diet (See Fig. 3.2).[151] Dr. Campbell permitted these privileges on the condition that patients would not abuse them. New conventions also included paying sums of money to 'hard-working and well-behaved lunatics'. In Bombay's asylums, superintendents also gave patients other incentives such as money for tobacco and small luxuries.[152] Patients displayed good behaviour in exchange for rewards, and doctors permitted this reward system to get patients to work. Each side engaged the other to 'achieve a specific end'.[153] Superintendents accommodated the practice of locals wanting to pay frequent visits to friends or relatives who were patients. Superintendents justified their negotiations with local practices based on perceptions of 'their partner's cultural premise'.[154] One superintendent asserted that he felt 'it is a duty to yield to the desires and demands of friends'.[155] The practice of permitting relatives to visit at any time, at the discretion of the superintendent, was included as part of the 'Rules for the Bombay Lunatic Asylum' drafted in 1864.[156] Asylum staff also permitted patients to visit relatives and to 'spend a day in the bazar'. They even allowed convalescents to go out on probation.[157] In 1883, one European ex-patient complained that asylum staff permitted paying convalescent patients to go out on walks with a keeper almost 'every evening' and one patient, he observed, was even allowed to go out with his brother.[158] Superintendents were willing to negotiate asylum practices to make the asylum more appealing to the local community.

While superintendents were willing to negotiate, they also expressed concern over other aspects of the asylum that they perceived as ill-suited to Indians. The architecture of asylum buildings was felt to be 'ill-calculated to meet the prejudices of caste and other peculiarities of native patients, and ill-suited for the Indian climate'.[159] F.S. Arnott, the Inspector

[151] This practice was also included in the Lunacy Act of 1858. Lunacy Act XXXVI of 1858, GoB, GD, 1862–1864/15, MSA.

[152] The system of rewarding patients was practised in Cowasji Jehangir Lunatic Asylum, Hyderabad, for some years. From the Surgeon General with the Government of Bombay to the Secretary of the Government of Bombay, 12 July 1901, GoB, GD, 1901/66, MSA.

[153] White, *The Middle Ground*, p. 51.

[154] Ibid., p. 52.

[155] Report on the Lunatic Asylum at Colaba for the Year Ending 1852, GoB, GD, 1853/48, MSA.

[156] Rules of the Bombay Lunatic Asylum, 1864, GoB, GD, 1862–1864/15, MSA.

[157] From the Superintendent, Lunatic Asylum, Colaba, to the Secretary to the Principal Inspector General, Medical Department, 31 July 1863, GoB, GD, 1862–1864/15, MSA.

[158] Letter to the Editor by a late patient, *Bombay Gazetteer*, 29 October 1863.

[159] From the Superintendent, Lunatic Asylum, Colaba, to the Secretary to the Principal Inspector General, Medical Department, 31 July 1863, GoB, GD, 1862–1864/15, MSA.

General of Hospitals, affirmed the same principles of accommodating Indian feelings and habits in his report on the site for a new central asylum. He stated 'that in deciding the location the feelings and even prejudices of friends must be treated with delicacy nor should the feelings of the patients be overlooked ... to the domestic habits of Natives, their love of home, their dread of separation ... and exile'.[160] Asylum buildings became an important symbol of negotiation between the local and colonial agencies.

Compared to asylums in other presidencies, Bombay's asylums represented a far more negotiated space between colonial agencies and local communities.[161] In 1880, the *Rast Goftar* condemned the government for trying to shift the Colaba Lunatic Asylum to the Byculla Club, as the locality was unhygienic, and what was 'unhealthy for Europeans cannot but prove equally detrimental to the health of lunatics'.[162] The government heeded this demand and the asylum was not moved. The Colaba Asylum housed both European and Indian patients and at its closure, asylum agencies shifted both groups of patients to the asylum at Yerawada.[163] Monetary contributions made to the asylum from affluent Hindu and Parsi families made it easier for them to negotiate asylum practices.[164] While superintendents continued to negotiate with local communities, they did not always agree with government policies regarding mental health treatment.

By the early twentieth century, superintendent's connectedness towards the Indians slowly turned into a rejection of western psychiatry as a

---

[160] From the Inspector General of Hospitals to the Secretary to the Principal Inspector General, Medical Department, Poona, 27 September 1864, GoB, GD, 1862–1864/15, MSA.

[161] Bhattacharyya argued that superintendents increasingly dictated the community's interaction with internal asylum practices. See Bhattacharyya, 'Indian Insanes, Lunacy in the "Native" Asylums of Colonial India', p. 211.

[162] RNP, *Rast Goftar*, 9 May 1880, K 4091-D, PG 1–444, GoB, MSA. The *Rast Goftar* was an Anglo-Gujarati weekly started in 1851 by Dadabhai Naoroji.

[163] All Indians except the Parsis were moved in 1902 to the lunatic asylum at Thana. Triennial Report on the Lunatic Asylums in the Bombay Presidency, 1912–1914, p. 1, NLS.

[164] Sir Cowasji Jehangir funded (Rs. 50,000) the building of the Hyderabad asylum completed in 1871; see A.W. Hughes, *A Gazetteer of the Province of Sindh* (London: George Bell and Sons, 1874), p. 206. Mr. Bhagwandas Narotamdas donated funds for the asylum in Thana; Vesting Order, The Charitable Endowment Act 1890, 18 August 1911, by L. Robertson, Secretary to the Government, GoB, GD, 1913/99, MSA. The Petit family, an elite Parsi family (N.M. Petit Trust) donated Rs. 20,000 for Parsi patients at the new central asylum in Yerawada; From C.F. Petit to the Secretary to the Government of Bombay, 24 January 1902, GoB, GD, 1902/61, MSA.

treatment method for 'Indian lunatics'. Superintendents declared that the colonial institution of asylum was not in need of 'an expert from England', but rather someone with 'experience' of Indian patients.[165] Superintendent Lt. Col. J.W.T. Anderson of Ahmedabad asserted that this person should be an officer from the IMS 'with experience of the habits and customs of the Natives of India, and not a novice from England with impracticable ideas as to the needs of Indian lunatics'. Because 'an expert from England without Indian experience' would fail, and the 'the innovations introduced in the first five years of his service would probably require undoing later on when he acquired the necessary local experience'.[166] Even the policies of the Sanitary Commission reflected the changing perceptions towards the effectiveness of western medicine and treatment in the Indian setting. Harcourt Butler, who presided over the Indian Sanitary Conference in 1911, recognized the inability of western methods to 'produce identical results in India'.[167] Superintendent Grayfoot reiterated the same beliefs regarding the application of western psychiatry in the Indian asylum, arguing that 'the conditions in India and Europe are so different for the uninitiated to understand that what is suitable for Europeans is not required in native asylums'.[168] Bombay's superintendents gradually began to consider western psychiatry ineffective in the treatment of Indian patients. They began to advocate the 'common-sense' treatment of Indian lunacy,[169] 'mutually invented'[170] by them and their subordinate staff. The superintendents felt that the 'present craze for experts' to treat Indian lunacy was

[165] From B.B. Grayfoot, Superintendent, Lunatic Asylum, Dharwar, to the Personal Asst. to the Surgeon General with the Government of Bombay, 10 August 1904, GoB, GD, 1907/81, MSA; From Lt. Col. J W T Anderson, Superintendent, Lunatic Asylum, Ahmedabad, to the Personal Asst. to the Surgeon General with the Government of Bombay, 10 July 1904, GoB, GD, 1907/81, MSA.

[166] From Lt. Col. J W T Anderson, Superintendent, Lunatic Asylum, Ahmedabad, to the Personal Asst. to the Surgeon General with the Government of Bombay, 10 July 1904, GoB, GD 1907/81, MSA.

[167] RNP, *Bombay Samachar*, 17 and 18 November 1911, in Mridula Ramanna, 'Perception of Sanitation and Medicine in Bombay, 1900–1914', in Tine and Mann, *Colonialism as Civilising Mission*, p. 222.

[168] From B.B. Grayfoot, Superintendent, Lunatic Asylum, Dharwar, to the Personal Asst. to the Surgeon General with the Government of Bombay, 10 August 1904, GoB, GD, 1907/81, MSA.

[169] From B.B. Grayfoot, Superintendent, Lunatic Asylum, Dharwar, to the Personal Asst. to the Surgeon General with the Government of Bombay, 10 August 1904, GoB, GD, 1907/81, MSA.

[170] White, *The Middle Ground*, p. 50.

'wholly unnecessary',[171] as the 'common-sense' treatment of Indian insanity was a method acceptable to patients, familiar to subordinate staff, convenient for superintendents, and inexpensive for the government. Colonial
superintendents claimed that European experts, nurses, and methods were
a waste of money for 'Indian lunatics'. The specialist would not even be
able to communicate with Indian patients whose languages it would take
'six years to learn' and at the end of that time, he would have to 'go home
to refer to his theories'. If a specialist from home was appointed to manage
asylums in India, he had to be someone with knowledge of 'India and
natives and had specialised lunacy as a hobby'.[172]

In 1914, Dr. W.S. Jagoe Shaw, Superintendent of the new lunatic asylum at Yerawada, attempted to change direction and to align Bombay's
colonial asylum with its European counterparts, based on the principles of
western psychiatry. Having worked in the asylums in Punjab, Lahore, and
Rangoon, he felt the need to reform the asylum system to re-establish
colonial hegemony within asylums. A staunch loyalist to western psychiatry and colonialism, Dr. Shaw clashed with most superintendents, not only
in the Bombay Presidency but also all over the Indian colony as he
attempted to change the designation 'lunatic asylum' to 'mental asylum'.
Superintendents argued that asylums were merely places of detention[173]
and 'could not be considered hospitals, as no lunatics ever recovered!'.[174]
Dr. Shaw ridiculed his opponents labelling them 'non-specialists'. He
finally succeeded, after five years, to bring about the change in the nomenclature with the support of the Director General of the IMS.[175] However,
the renaming did not ensure a change in the nature and extent of use of
asylums, as he noted that the 'the chief obstruction to the progress of
psychiatry in India ... was the absence of a definitely expressed public

[171] From B.B. Grayfoot, Superintendent, Lunatic Asylum, Dharwar, to the Personal Asst.
to the Surgeon General with the Government of Bombay, 10 August 1904, GoB, GD,
1907/81, MSA; From Lt. Col. J.W.T. Anderson, Superintendent, Lunatic Asylum,
Ahmedabad, to the Personal Asst. to the Surgeon General with the Government of Bombay,
10 July 1904, GoB, GD, 1907/81, MSA.

[172] From B.B. Grayfoot, Superintendent, Lunatic Asylum, Dharwar, to the Personal Asst.
to the Surgeon General with the Government of Bombay, 10 August 1904, GoB, GD,
1907/81, MSA.

[173] From the Superintendent, Central Lunatic Asylum, Yerawada, to the Surgeon General
with the Government of Bombay, GoB, GD, 1922/ 2257-B, MSA.

[174] Shaw, 'The Alienist Department', p. 339.

[175] Ibid., pp. 338–339.

opinion' and the 'preference of Ayurvedic and indigenous systems to ... modern methods of treatment'.[176]

Superintendents as colonial agents failed to establish hegemony in Bombay's asylums. Historians have argued that by the early decades of the twentieth century the Indian 'native' lunatic asylums were transformed into 'bastions of colonial hegemony'.[177] However, Bombay's lunatic asylums clearly deviated from this model. Colonial agencies failed to establish hegemony because of the shortage of staff[178] and finances, which meant that superintendents had to continue to negotiate with staff and local communities. Up until the 1930s, superintendents relied on local donations for amusement facilities for patients.[179] The Ranchi Indian Mental Hospital was an exception, where, under the superintendence of Dr. Dhunjibhoy, a Parsi doctor, the hospital transformed into a colonial 'archetype'.[180] Criticizing his predecessors, he faithfully executed tasks of surveillance and discipline, maintenance of a productive patient class, and production of the knowledge of Indian insanity.[181] By 1930, Superintendent Dhunjibhoy had started using contemporary treatment methods practised around the world. His strong adherence to western psychiatry stemmed from the fact that he wanted to establish himself in the colonial medical hierarchy. Faced with competition and racial discrimination from his European counterparts, his propagation of western methods of treatment gave him a professional edge over them.[182] Despite the progress made

---

[176] Ibid., p. 334.

[177] Ibid., p. 211.

[178] Annual Reports on Mental Hospitals in the Bombay Presidency (AR) for the Year 1933, p. 7, NLS.

[179] AR, 1933, p. 7.

[180] Bhattacharyya, 'Indian Insanes, Lunacy in the "Native" Asylums of Colonial India', p. iii.

[181] Dr. Dhunjibhoy stated: 'With the progress of civilization, India, like Europe began to erect grim, sombre buildings ... the old asylums were manned by brutal types of attendants, who were ready to impose manacles and chains and stripes at their own free will'. Dr. Dhunjibhoy displays a colonial self-understanding in criticizing the asylum system and subordinate attendants. A strong advocate for western psychiatry, he produced knowledge about Indian insanity fulfilling the expectation of the colonial state. See Jal Eduji Dhunjibhoy, 'A Brief Resume of the Types of Insanity Commonly Met with in India, with a Full Description of the "Indian Hemp Insanity" Peculiar to the Country', *British Journal of Psychiatry*, Vol. 76, April 1930, pp. 254–264.

[182] Waltraud Ernst, 'The Indianization of Colonial Medicine: The Case of Psychiatry in the Early-Twentieth-Century British India', *NTM International Journal of History & Ethics of Natural Sciences, Technology and Medicine*, Vol. 20, May 2012, p. 63.

with treatment methods in the Ranchi Hospital, the Ranchi experiment could not be repeated anywhere in the Bombay asylums.

CONCLUSION

The European superintendent as the backbone of the asylum hierarchy failed in disseminating the knowledge and practice of western psychiatry. Limited by stringent budgets, constant scrutiny, and power contestation within the colonial bureaucracy, European superintendents devised their own ways of managing and treating Indian patients. The superintendents' failure to execute surveillance and discipline, produce knowledge, and maintain a productive patient class meant that colonial hegemony evaded Bombay's asylums. Internal power contestations affected the functioning of the asylum system, causing its failure.

The failure of the agency of the superintendents facilitated the creation of what we have called here the 'middle ground'. Superintendents began to assert their expertise in Indian insanity by devising new strategies to continue their agency. Superintendents, asylum staff, local communities, and patients negotiated asylum practices. Gradually, over the nineteenth and early twentieth centuries, superintendents distanced themselves from western psychiatry as a method of treatment for Indian insanity and displayed an increasing connectedness to hybridized methods of treatment within the asylum. Bombay's superintendents resigned to running the asylum and managing their patients through 'common-sense' treatment. The nature of the asylum as a middle ground irked the government, but for superintendents, the creation of the middle ground was both necessary and inevitable.

CHAPTER 4

The 'Common-Sense' Treatment of Indian Insanity

In India, we do not pretend to be experts but treat lunacy in a common-sense way; our methods are the same and our results I think, just as good.[1]

In 1904, Superintendent Grayfoot rejected a government proposal for bringing in a specialist to manage the Bombay asylums. He strongly believed that while psychiatry appeared to make progress, those who claimed to be specialists in lunacy had only provided a more complex classification of mental illness. Treatment in England, he stated, merely included 'treating symptoms, gentle discipline and good nursing'.[2] Grayfoot and other superintendents in Bombay believed that the hybrid[3] treatment methods combining western psychiatry and Indian practices,

[1] From B.B. Grayfoot, Superintendent, Lunatic Asylum, Dharwar, to the Personal Asst. to the Surgeon General with the Government of Bombay, 10 August 1904, GoB, GD, 1907/81, MSA, Mumbai.

[2] From B.B. Grayfoot, Superintendent, Lunatic Asylum, Dharwar, to the Personal Asst. to the Surgeon General with the Government of Bombay, 10 August 1904, GoB, GD, 1907/81, MSA.

[3] Waltraud Ernst and Anouska Bhattacharyya identified the hybrid nature of the colonial asylum. See Waltraud Ernst, 'Idioms of Madness and Colonial Boundaries: The Case of the European and "Native" Mentally Ill in Early Nineteenth-Century British India', *Comparative Studies in Society and History*, Vol. 39, No. 01, January 1997, p. 168; Anouska Bhattacharyya, 'Indian Insanes, Lunacy in the "Native" Asylums of Colonial India, 1858–1912', PhD Thesis, Harvard University, 2013, p. 75.

© The Author(s) 2018
S. A. Pinto, *Lunatic Asylums in Colonial Bombay*,
Mental Health in Historical Perspective,
https://doi.org/10.1007/978-3-319-94244-5_4

invented in Bombay's asylums, were the most effective way of regulating and maintaining their asylums. Hybrid treatment practices that superintendents advocated were a 'common-sense' way of treating Indian patients. It ideally involved clothing, feeding, treating the body of the patients, and providing amusement and occupation. As one superintendent explained:

> The native lunatic wants to be well-clothed, fed, treated when ill, amused in airy day wards, to be occupied in a garden and allowed to see his friends and have much freedom as possible; to have attendants who speak his language and understand his ways.[4]

Colonial and Indian encounters within and circumstances outside the asylum were the cause of such hybrid treatment regimes. Hybridity in the practice of western medical treatment in India was a necessity 'in order to gain social and cultural respectability'.[5] Such hybrid treatment practices, however, irrespective of the intention of the asylum medical class and staff, often led to the undermining of Indian social and cultural norms. This chapter argues, then, that the 'common-sense' treatment of patients, because of its hybrid nature, considerably influenced the use of the asylum.

On one hand, hybrid treatment practices challenged the superiority of western medicine and exposed its 'relative ineffectiveness'. In relation to other bodily diseases, European doctors 'even when conspicuously borrowing from indigenous practice ... remained... disposed to believe in the superiority of their own methods and medicine'.[6] However, with mental health treatment, European asylum superintendents themselves began to challenge the efficacy of western treatment practices and actively resisted them. The subordinate staff and European superintendents both actively participated in the subversion of western psychiatric practice. The asylum, envisioned as the 'citadel'[7] of colonialism because of its hybrid treatment practices, became a sinister effigy of the colonial state. While colonial

---

[4] From B.B. Grayfoot, Superintendent, Lunatic Asylum, Dharwar, to the Personal Asst. to the Surgeon General with the Government of Bombay, 10 August 1904, GoB, GD, 1907/81, MSA.

[5] David Arnold, *Colonizing the Body: State Medicine and Epidemic Disease in Nineteenth-Century India* (Berkley and California: University of California Press, 1993), p. 251.

[6] Arnold, *Colonizing the Body*, p. 181.

[7] Ernst, 'Idioms of Madness and Colonial Boundaries', p. 172.

agencies still used the asylum to execute the 'cultural project of control',[8] they never achieved complete hegemony.

On the other hand, hybrid treatment practices set limits to resistance to colonial control. Ashish Nandy argued that the 'ultimate violence' of colonialism was that it paradoxically challenged the colonized to contest it, and yet simultaneously set the 'psychological limits' for such resistance.[9] Hybridity, then, the chapter argues, was a means of setting psychological boundaries within which patients could express their Indian self-consciousness, as a sign of resistance. The superintendent and asylum staff, however, predetermined the boundaries for expressing such resistance.

Hybridity manifested in two ways: through the inclusion of local practices or medicines, and the adoption of western psychiatry to local conditions. In 1853, Dr. Campbell described asylum treatment practices in two broad categories: hygiene and moral treatment. Hygiene treatment included 'airing, clothing, bathing and feeding' and moral treatment included 'amusement and exercise' (labour).[10] This chapter focuses on the three most extensively applied treatment methods in Bombay's asylums: clothing, diet, and occupation. In clothing and diet treatment, hybridity was manifest in permitting Indian garments and food. Superintendents also hybridized occupation to suit local conditions. In Bombay, hygiene treatment remained the main method of treating patients for the first half of the century. Moral treatment administered through occupation was more extensively used with diet and clothing only after the mid-nineteenth century.

CLOTHING AS TREATMENT

In the colonial asylum, the asylum staff used clothing to colonize and civilize. Clothing had different connotations in Bombay's asylums compared to Victorian asylums where doctors used clothing as a 'means of recovery and a reward' for asylum patients.[11] Michael Dietler argued that clothing

[8] Nicholas Dirks, 'Foreword', in Bernard Cohn, *Colonialism and its Forms of Knowledge: The British in India* (New Jersey: Princeton University Press, 1996), p. ix.

[9] Ashish Nandy, *The Intimate Enemy: Loss and Recovery of Self Under Colonialism* (Delhi: Oxford University Press, 1983), p. 3.

[10] Report on the Lunatic Asylum at Colaba for the Year Ending 1852, GoB, GD, 1853/48, MSA.

[11] Vivienne Richmond, *Clothing the Poor in Nineteenth-Century England* (Cambridge: Cambridge University Press, 2013), p. 269.

played an important role in the colonial context. European missionaries used it to 'colonize the consciousness' as well as to train indigenous peoples in ideals of 'work discipline, temporality and gender relations'.[12] In the colonies, colonizers used clothing or the lack of it as a measuring tool on a civilizational scale. Since Indian nakedness was interpreted as 'primitiveness',[13] clothing patients in the asylum was a way medical and asylum staff executed and lived the 'fantasy of the civilizing mission'.[14] Indian nakedness for the colonial government was a threat to 'colonial dignity, control and orderliness'.[15] Clothing was an integral part of asylum treatment, since the British believed that 'colonial nakedness was potentially dangerous … but also tameable'.[16] Clothing as therapy, then, involved civilizing Indian patients by properly covering them and thus restoring 'dignity, control and orderliness'.[17]

Colonial agencies interpreted nakedness and semi-nakedness as symptoms of madness. Asylum doctors and civil surgeons often issued medical certificates stating refusal to wear clothing or the tearing of clothing as indications of insanity. In 1814, Dr. Maxwell, Superintendent of the Colaba Lunatic Asylum, reported three patient-clothing encounters. The first patient, Shaik Ahmed, he stated, 'refused to put on clean clothing' and even 'tore them to shreds'. The second patient, Mohammed Ali, was so violent that 'it was impossible to keep clothing on him'. A few months later Dr. Maxwell noted how Ali had a 'dislike for clothing and hospital attendants'. The third patient was a woman named Joaquina who 'twice has torn her cloaths [sic] … she likes much to be naked it is with difficulty

[12] Michael Dietler, 'Culinary Encounters: Food, Identity and Colonialism', in Katheryn C. Twiss (ed.), *The Archaeology of Food and Identity* (Carbondale: Southern Illinois University Press, 2007), p. 228.

[13] Mouloud Siber and Bouteldja Riche, 'The Aesthetic of Natives' Dress and Undress: Colonial Stereotype and Mimicry in Paul Gauguin's and William Somerset Maugham's Cultural Forms', *Linguistic Practices,* Vol. 19, 2013, p. 27; Philippa Levine, 'States of Undress: Nakedness and the Colonial Imagination', *Victorian Studies,* Vol. 50, No. 2, 2008, p. 189.

[14] James Mills, '"More Important to Civilise than Subdue"? Lunatic Asylums, Psychiatric Practice and Fantasies of the "Civilising Mission" in British India 1858–1900', in Harald Fischer-Tiné and Michael Mann (eds.), *Colonialism as Civilising Mission* (London: Anthem Press, 2003), pp. 171–182.

[15] Rianne Siebenga, 'Colonial India's "Fanatical Fakirs" and their Popular Representations', *History and Anthropology,* Vol. 23, No. 4, 2012, p. 449.

[16] Levine, 'States of Undress', p. 210.

[17] Ibid., p. 210.

that she can be kept clothed'.[18] Even in the late nineteenth century, colonial agencies deduced that a person's attitude to clothing indicated his mental condition. Certificates issued to patients Haridas Naranjan, Narayan Gunja, and Dundoo stated how they 'tore every bit of cloth', showed 'a neglect of clothing',[19] and refused to cover even 'private parts carefully'.[20] The *fakir*,[21] in particular, embodied 'disorder and madness'[22] because of his 'partial nakedness'[23] and his sale and use of *charas* (a type of hemp).[24] A 'lapse of modesty'[25] in clothing was a symptom of madness, and asylum staff treated it by properly clothing patients.

While colonial agencies perceived Indian nakedness as madness, it had different implications based on gender. Doctors adopted Victorian perceptions of the links between indigenous male nakedness and violence[26] and female nakedness and promiscuity in the diagnosis and treatment of patients in Bombay. They described male patients who refused to wear clothing as having symptoms that were more violent, as exemplified in the cases of Shaik and Ali. Surgeon Maxwell interpreted Joaquina's refusal to dress as evidence of her promiscuity; he elucidated that she 'liked to be naked'. Joaquina, prior to her admission, was pregnant out of wedlock; Dr. Maxwell used her preference for nakedness as evidence of her promiscuity, and he concluded her promiscuity was a symptom of her madness. In 1853, Dr. Campbell reported that a majority of the women in his asylum were of 'low caste' and had led 'vicious profligate lives' and 'their

[18] From Asst. Surgeon J.A. Maxwell to the Chief Secretary to the Government of Bombay, 4 June 1814, GoB, PDD, 1814/368, MSA.

[19] From R.C. Candy Esquire, Magistrate of Kanara, to the Secretary, Judicial Department, Government of Bombay, 11 June 1881, GoB, GD, 1881/56, MSA.

[20] Medical Certificate Issued by A. Pereira, Civil Surgeon, 16 August 1881, GoB, GD, 1881/56, MSA.

[21] Beggars, *fakirs*, and mendicants accounted for more than 70 per cent of the asylum population in the Presidency. APR, 1880, NLS, p. 2.

[22] Nile Green, 'Breaking the Begging Bowl: Morals, Drugs, and Madness in the Fate of the Muslim Faqir', *South Asian History and Culture*, Vol. 5, No. 2, 2014, p. 237.

[23] Siebenga, 'Colonial India's "Fanatical Fakirs"', p. 449.

[24] Ibid.; Green, 'Breaking the Begging Bowl', p. 237.

[25] A medical form mentions the 'lapse of modesty' as a symptom of Pandu Dadji's insanity. Form C, Mode of Taking Notes in a Case of Insanity before Sending a Patient to the Asylum, 23 June 1881, GoB, GD, 1881/56, MSA.

[26] Levine argued that in the colonial imagination, indigenous male nakedness was linked to 'physical danger' and female nakedness was perceived as 'sexual availability'. See Philippa Levine, 'Naked Truths: Bodies, Knowledge, and the Erotics of Colonial Power', *Journal of British Studies*, Vol. 52, Iss. 1, 2013, pp. 16–18.

symptoms are generally such as might be expected to ensure on a course of dissipation and debauchery'.[27] One female patient's medical certificate noted the 'tearing of clothes' as one of the 'Facts determining insanity'; the certificate also recorded that she was a registered prostitute.[28] Doctors interpreted a patient's refusal to wear clothing as a sign of morbidity, and clothing became a way of civilizing the savage—the violent Indian man and the promiscuous Indian woman. Clothing treatment included several steps.

The first step involved bathing and examining the patient. Madness provided unrestricted access to the body of the patient. The Preamble of the Poona Asylum noted that patients were to be 'washed as soon as possible prior to the necessary clothing being given to them'.[29] Asylum doctors examined the 'native body' for the 'purposes of knowledge'.[30] Mental illness became a legitimate excuse to survey, examine, and classify Indian bodies, since to 'unclothe was to uncover the truth about the native'.[31]

> Observing the uncovered body, not for aesthetic but scientific purposes could simultaneously indicate control over the body observed, a panoptical manoeuvre that signalled colonial possession, colonial knowledge and colonial desire.[32]

On the pretext of examination or treatment, asylum staff undressed and observed patients several times. The observation of the Indian body was part of the diagnostic process. In colonial asylums, Mills argued that the body was the omphalos of the diagnostic process.[33] Examination of patient bodies included examining genitalia. In 1814, Surgeon Maxwell treated Balloo, a patient, for 'anasarca in the penis' by slightly puncturing the skin. In another patient, he noted 'swelling in the right testicle'. He also stated that he had not found the cause of the swelling, indicating further

---

[27] Report on the Lunatic Asylum at Colaba for the Year Ending 1852, GoB, GD, 1853/48, MSA.

[28] Form A, Certificate of Medical Officer, GoB, GD, 1885/73, MSA.

[29] Rules of the Poona Lunatic Asylum, Preamble, 1874, GoB, GD, 1874/32, MSA.

[30] Levine, 'States of Undress', p. 209.

[31] Ibid., p. 199.

[32] Ibid., p. 207.

[33] James Mills, 'The Lunatic Asylum in British India, 1857 to 1880: Colonialism, Medicine and Power', PhD Thesis, The University of Edinburgh, 1997, pp. 33–40.

examination to diagnose the cause of the swelling.[34] Levine argued that the need to identify differences between the races and to provide evidence against the genesis story of 'origin from a common stock' motivated the obsession with examining genitalia.[35] Once bathed, examined, and classified, patients were then dressed.

The asylum staff assigned the label of 'treatment' to clothing, since they perceived Indian nakedness as a symptom of madness. In the first half of the nineteenth century, asylum inspection reports focused on four aspects of asylum treatment, which included 'clothing, cleanliness, diet and medical treatment'.[36] In the mid-1800s, Superintendent Campbell reported the treatment of Indian patients with clothing. Dr. John Conolly's ideas had greatly influenced Dr. Campbell, who emphasized the need for clean, tidy, and appropriate clothing for men and women in the asylum.[37] In the Annual Asylum Report for 1852, Dr. Campbell listed asylum clothing given to patients at the Colaba Lunatic Asylum:

4 Cotton *Dhoties* [garment which is worn on the lower body],
2 White *Pugdies* [also *Pugris*: turban/headgear],
4 Ditto *Cholnas* [kind of short breeches],[38]
4 Ditto *Langorties* [underwear for the lower body],
4 Ditto Double *Bundies* [inner wear for upper body, similar to a vest],
4 Ditto *Cumblies* [also *Kumblies*: rough woollen blankets].[39]

The items of clothing listed by Dr. Campbell were essential parts of the asylum clothing practice even in the latter half of the nineteenth century;

[34] From Asst. Surgeon J.A. Maxwell to the Chief Secretary to the Government of Bombay, 4 June 1814, GoB, PDD, 1814/368, MSA.

[35] Levine, 'States of Undress', p. 207.

[36] From the Senior Magistrate of Police and President of the Medical Board to the President and Governor in Council, Mounstuart Elphinstone, 1 September 1821, GoB, GD, 1821–1823/24/27, MSA; From the Member of the Medical Board to the President and Governor in Council Mounstuart Elphinstone, 1 February 1824, GoB, GD, 1824/10/66, MSA.

[37] Conolly emphasized the importance of clothing as part of the asylum regime. He explained: 'In regulating the dress of insane patients as in every regulation for them we consider not only its first and indispensable uses, but also its effects on the mind'. See John Conolly, *The Construction and Government of Lunatic Asylums as Hospitals for the Insanes* (London: John Church Hill, 1847), p. 63.

[38] Superintendent of the Lunatic Asylum at Poona to the Secretary to the Surgeon General with the Government of Bombay, 1 December 1883, GoB, GD, 1883/95, MSA.

[39] Report on the Lunatic Asylum at Colaba for the Year Ending 1852, GoB, GD, 1853/48, MSA.

however, the medical class had made a few more additions to asylum attire to appropriately clothe the 'native'. During this time, the attire for male patients included jackets, dungarees, drawers, caps, *dhoties*, and *pugries*. Asylum staff provided female patients with sarees and *choolies*.[40] Furthermore, footwear was part of the asylum uniform; these included 'sandals or *chappals* (slippers)'. Asylum staff used canvas frocks as a restraint for destructive patients.[41]

Asylum staff administered clothing treatment appropriately keeping in mind gender, class, and race. Climate also influenced quality and quantity of asylum clothing. While appropriating clothing, however, they did not make caste distinctions. Asylum clothing varied in different asylums of the Presidency. In Hyderabad, '*Peranas*,[42] Pyjamas and Caps' were used for patients. Classification of uniforms in Ahmedabad was based on sex. Asylum uniforms included drawers and jackets for men, '*Cholies, geegras* and *sadees*' for women.[43] In Dharwar, men were clothed in more layers than women. Men's asylum uniform consisted of 'Bundees, Cholnas, Langoorties, Caps and Kumblies', while the uniform for female patients included 'choolies and sarees'. At the Poona Lunatic Asylum, the uniform consisted of *bundees, cholnas*, drawers, *dhoties, langorties, pugries*, and sarees. In Poona, clothing was made of three types of fabric: double dungaree, looie, and cotton. In Colaba, uniforms for European patients consisted of banians, caps, drawers, shirts, hats (Pith or Felt), socks, boots, and slippers. The asylum also provided European patients with nightgowns. European and Eurasian females were given extra chemises and petticoats. Asylum staff at Colaba assigned Indian patients with uniforms similar to the ones used in Poona; furthermore, at Colaba distinction was made between lower- and high-class Indian patients[44] and Parsis. Superintendents preferred 'coarser clothing' for Indian patients, since they were stronger and better adopted to maintain the orderliness of the asylum.[45] The Asylum Rules of the Presidency made a special provision for

---

[40] *Choolies* is the plural form of *Choli*, a blouse or bodice worn with a saree or *lehenga* (a type of skirt).

[41] From the Civil Surgeon, Ratnagiri, to the Secretary to the Surgeon General with the Government of Bombay, 28 February 1886, GoB, GD, 1886/58, MSA.

[42] *Perana* is a type of shirt.

[43] *Geegra* is a long skirt worn under a saree; *sadees* is the same as sarees.

[44] Asylum General Rules (Bombay Presidency) submitted with Letter 1103 from the Surgeon General, IMD, 13 April 1874, GD, 1874/32, MSA.

[45] APR, 1875, p. 25, NLS.

Parsi patients, by additionally providing them with '*sudras*[46] of fine cloth'. Apart from clothing, only the Colaba Lunatic Asylum provided patients with footwear. Footwear for Europeans and 'natives' of a 'better class' included canvas shoes and slippers, while the asylum provided other Indian patients with 'native' shoes.[47] The distinctions made in uniform and footwear between 'better class' and other patients display the intent of asylum doctors to make the colonial lunatic asylum a place for patients of all classes. While asylum agencies maintained class distinctions in clothing, asylum uniforms simultaneously homogenized Indian patients.

Uniformity in clothing provides evidence of the civilizing mission. On one hand, the colonial asylum uniform had a 'homogenizing intent'.[48] On the other, it reflected ideas of 'separateness from the Indian population' that the British sought to establish by encouraging Indian people to dress in an 'oriental manner'.[49] In the mid-nineteenth century, Dr. Campbell clothed all his male patients with the same Indian attire of *dhoti*, *pugdi*, and *cholna* without caste or religious considerations.[50] Patients had to wear inner and outer garments. In Bombay's asylums, doctors maintained uniformity even in colour. In contrast, Victorian asylums gave patients a choice to choose certain 'colours and styles for hats and handkerchiefs'.[51] Dress served as an incentive, and doctors recommended the introduction of variety rather than absolute uniformity. All patients, except for a few who had their own clothes, both men and women, were dressed in white. In India, colours had varied meanings based on caste and *varna* (social class) and the 'hierarchy of colour symbolism', and they varied for men and women.[52] The colour white in Indian society implied a 'cooling effect'.[53] The colour white, from the colonial perspective, was the suitable

---

[46] *Sudra* is a sacred muslin undershirt worn by the Parsis.

[47] Asylum General Rules (Bombay Presidency) submitted with Letter 1103 from the Surgeon General, IMD, 13 April 1874, GD, 1874/32, MSA.

[48] Richmond, *Clothing the Poor in Nineteenth-Century England*, pp. 268, 283.

[49] Cohn, *Colonialism and its Forms of Knowledge*, p. 121; Emma Tarlo, *Clothing Matters: Dress and Identity in India* (Chicago: University of Chicago Press, 1996), p. 13.

[50] Report on the Lunatic Asylum at Colaba for the Year Ending 1852, GoB, GD, 1853/48, MSA.

[51] Richmond, *Clothing the Poor*, p. 268.

[52] Catherine Weiberger Thomas, *Ashes of Immortality: Widow Burning in India*, trans. Jeffrey Mehlman and David Gordon White (Chicago: University of Chicago Press, 1999), p. 24.

[53] Brenda E.F. Beck, 'Colour and Heat in South Indian Ritual', *Man*, New Series, Vol. 4, No. 4, December 1969, p. 559.

colour for clothing Indian men as a way of calming the 'savage' Indian male. Among Indian women, white denoted 'chastity and virtue'.[54] Dressing Indian women in white was a way of taming her promiscuity, inducing in her a sense of morality, and preserving her chastity.

The asylum uniform helped maintain order and cleanliness. The Asylum General Rules in 1874 upheld Dr. Campbell's clothing list for male patients. The Rules initially permitted female patients to dress according to their 'caste and former mode of life'.[55] In 1907, however, the government revised the Rules and removed the exemption made for female patients. The principle of cleanliness became the criteria for appropriate clothing in the asylum, as the Rules did not permit patients to wear 'dirty clothes'.[56] Since most patients were from 'poorer classes',[57] this rule only reinforced the use of asylum uniforms. The insistence on uniformity in Bombay's asylums contrasted the liberality of dress permitted in Victorian asylums. The process of appropriately dressing patients in Bombay's asylums was a far more rigid process than in Britain and asylum staff closely supervised it.

Clothing treatment involved the engagement of the agency of both asylum staff and patients. The superintendent had the authority to monitor clothing and supply it according to his discretion, depending on 'peculiarities, position, character and symptoms'[58] of patients. The senior attendant of the ward was responsible for the cleanliness and tidiness of patients and their clothing. The head attendant and overseer were responsible for maintaining an inventory of 'clothing and other articles in his ward'. Attendants had to 'use their utmost endeavours to prevent the destruction and defilement of clothing'.[59] The asylum maintained a daily

---

[54] Sarah Lamb, 'Aging, Gender and Widowhood: Perspectives from Rural West Bengal', *Contributions to Indian Sociology*, Vol. 33, No 3, 1999, p. 546; Uma Chakravarti, 'Ageing, Gender Caste and Labour: Ideological and Material Structure of Widowhood', *Economic and Political Weekly*, Vol. 30, No. 36, 9 September 1995, p. 2251.

[55] Asylum General Rules (Bombay Presidency) submitted with Letter 1103 from the Surgeon General, IMD, 13 April 1874, GD, 1874/32, MSA.

[56] Rules for the Lunatic Asylums in the Bombay Presidency (Up to 1907), GoB, GD, 1908/80, MSA.

[57] Asst. Surgeon, Colaba Lunatic Asylum, to the Secretary of the Medical Board, 21 February 1847, GoB, GD, 1847/ 41, MSA.

[58] Report on the Lunatic Asylum at Colaba for the Year Ending 1852, GoB, GD, 1853/48, MSA.

[59] Asylum General Rules (Bombay Presidency) submitted with Letter 1103 from the Surgeon General, IMD, 13 April 1874, GoB, GD, 1874/32, MSA.

list of clothing destroyed by patients. Colonial jails supplied Bombay's white asylum uniforms.[60] Towards the end of the century, however, super-intendents employed jail workers or tailors to train asylum patients in spin-ning. Eventually these patients manufactured their own clothing at asylum factories.[61] Superintendents thus successfully employed patients in the execution of their own clothing treatment.

The practice and the perception of clothing as treatment evolved over the nineteenth century. Negotiations over treatment practices between superintendents and asylum staff affected the notion of clothing as treat-ment. The increasing sense of commonality displayed by superintendents emerging from real encounters with Indians gradually changed the per-ceptions of Indian nakedness and primitiveness held on to by their other colonial counterparts. The Annual Asylum Report for 1895 credited the improvement in mortality rates at the Hyderabad Asylum to the willing-ness of patients to wear clothing:

> The improvement may also be attributed to some extent to the fact that inmates have been made to wear their clothing which they do now in most cases willingly. They are thus not so much exposed as they were in the previ-ous years.[62]

While clothing continued to be an integral part of asylum treatment in the early twentieth century, superintendents displayed a greater amount of leniency towards patients. Asylum rules specified that those patients who 'refused to wear clothing should not be compelled to do so', and patients who habitually refused clothing were allowed to be left in free cells or enclo-sures and provided with a mat to lie on.[63] Among the asylum staff, percep-tions of Indian attitudes towards clothing began to change as they projected clothing as the 'want' of the native patient.[64] As Superintendent Barry

---

[60] APR, 1875, p. 23, NLS.
[61] APR, 1897, p. 25; APR, 1898, p. 10; and Triennial Report on the Lunatic Asylums under the Government of Bombay, 1912–1914, p. 6, NLS.
[62] APR, 1895, p. 6, NLS.
[63] Rules for the Lunatic Asylums in the Bombay Presidency (Up to 1907), GoB, GD, 1908/80, MSA. The rules were based on Asylum Rules for 1874, and only a few minor changes were made to them. However, rules applying to clothing remained the same.
[64] From B.B. Grayfoot, Superintendent Lunatic Asylum, Dharwar, to the Personal Asst. to the Surgeon General with the Government of Bombay, 10 August 1904, GoB, GD, 1907/81, MSA.

suggested in 1904, the 'native lunatic wants to be well-clothed'.[65] Superintendents' letters depict Indian patients as preferring clothing rather than 'nakedness'. By the early twentieth century, a marked change is evident in the superintendent's perception of the Indian desire for clothing. Despite this change, the government continued to insist on the importance of clothing patients properly. In 1908, when an assessment of lunatic asylums in the Presidency was ordered, officers were expected to gather 'information of importance such as the treatment of patients who persisted in tearing their clothes and going naked, the arrangement of padded cells, employment of epileptics and isolation of phithisical cases'.[66] The colonial government continued to see Indian nakedness as a threat to colonial 'orderliness'[67] and therefore emphasized the need for monitoring clothing treatment.

Colonial asylum staff often engaged in inappropriate use of clothing in attempting to clothe the 'native' patient appropriately. Clothing was an integral part of the self-consciousness of various social and religious groups in India; few patients would have wanted to give up the attire they identified with.[68] Even though the patient seemed to have had the freedom to express his/her preference for Indian clothing, hybridity in clothing treatment set the 'psychological limits' for such expressions. Preconceived ideas about local people and economic expediency were the basis for negotiations on clothing treatment. Presumptions, for example, included beliefs that all Indian groups wore certain types of attire, like a *pugri*. Forcing patients to adopt inner and outer garments often went against their cultural preferences, since a change of clothes was akin to a 'change of cultural allegiance'.[69] Moreover, adopting white as the uniform colour, especially for female patients, was culturally inappropriate and insensitive, since in India only widows wore white.[70] While making distinctions in clothing for the favoured Parsi or occasionally between paying and non-paying patients, the asylum staff 'reduced vastly complex codes and their associated meanings to a few metonyms'.[71]

[65] From B.B. Grayfoot, Superintendent Lunatic Asylum, Dharwar, to the Personal Asst. to the Surgeon General with the Government of Bombay, 10 August 1904, GoB, GD, 1907/81, MSA.

[66] From the Surgeon General with the Government of Bombay to the Secretary to the Government of Bombay, 22 February 1909, GoB, GD, 1908/80, MSA.

[67] Siebenga, 'Colonial India's "Fanatical Fakirs"', p. 449.

[68] Tarlo, *Clothing Matters*, p. 24.

[69] Nirad Chaudhuri, *Culture in the Vanity Bag* (Bombay: Jaico, 1976), p. 73.

[70] Margaret Owen, *A World of Widows* (London: Zed Books, 1996), p. 17.

[71] Cohn, *Colonialism and its Forms of Knowledge*, p. 162.

Clothing treatment was an important tool in the maintenance and rein-forcement of distinction between the colonial and the colonized. The British had a 'psychological dependence' on clothing because it served to maintain their Englishness in the colony.[72] As asylum practices represented colonial-local relations, clothing treatment was the colonial way of assert-ing their own Englishness. Clothing treatment involved civilizing the Indian into an idealized colonial subject who was conscious of his other-ness and subservient to authority, rather than an 'idealized European who was productive, efficient, ordered and rational', as James Mills has argued.[73]

ASYLUM FOODSCAPES: DIET TREATMENT

Diet played a crucial role in treating Indian patients.[74] Diet as therapy was more than mere administration of food to patients. Food within the asylum had complex meanings. Michael Dielter, in his assessment of food, has argued that food as an 'embodiment of material culture' car-ries different implications based on its 'techniques of preparation, pat-terns of association and exclusion, modes of serving and consumption, [and] aesthetic evaluations'.[75] This section uses Dielter's framework to understand the connotation of food in the treatment of patients. In ana-lysing diet treatment in Bombay's lunatic asylums, this section examines four aspects of the material construction of food entailing production, preparation, consumption, and distribution. The limited number of treatment methods and the need for controlling the Indian body made medical staff have 'great faith in the curative agency of a good feeding'.[76] Superintendents believed that in order 'to restore the mind', they had to bring the 'physical frame of its inhabitants' into 'a sound and vigorous state'.[77] Asylum staff closely monitored patients through different pro-cesses of diet treatment. Bombay's asylum foodscapes reflected colonial

---

[72] Tarlo, *Clothing Matters*, p. 37.

[73] Mills argued that diet and occupation as part of asylum treatment was used to create an 'idealized European'. See James Mills, "'More Important to Civilise than Subdue'", p. 189.

[74] Shilpi Rajpal, 'Quotidian Madness: Time, Management and Asylums in Colonial North India', *Studies in History*, Vol. 31, No. 2, p. 221.

[75] Michael Dietler, 'Culinary Encounters', p. 222.

[76] Report on the Lunatic Asylum at Colaba for the Year Ending 1852, GoB, GD, 1853/48, MSA.

[77] From the Superintendent, Lunatic Asylum, Colaba, to the Secretary to the Medical Board, 21 June 1851, GoB, GD, 1851/15, MSA.

attitudes towards Indian society. The unequal distribution of food provides evidence of the infiltration of capitalist principles influencing the
asylum system.

Diet treatment began with production and preparation. Indian patients
were intimately involved in the two processes. Race and class determined
the extent of patient involvement in food production. Asylum staff did not
make Europeans, Eurasians, and paying patients labour for their food,[78]
while the Indian patients were involved in various ways in the production
of their own food. At the Ahmedabad Asylum, staff employed women to
grind grain.[79] At Dharwar and Ahmedabad, patients grew their vegetables.[80] Surgeon Major Keelan, Superintendent at the Sir Cowasji Jehangir
Asylum, Hyderabad, reported that patients worked under a *mali* (gardener) to ensure a supply of fresh vegetables daily. At the same asylum, the
superintendent gradually accustomed patients to the cooking room. He
employed them to do various tasks in the cooking room in 1873, and by
1885 male patients at Hyderabad were regularly cooking their food.[81]
Across the asylums of the Presidency, superintendents assigned the task of
grain grinding to female patients while they assigned men the cultivation
of vegetables and cooking. Once prepared, asylum staff meticulously
supervised the consumption of food by patients.

Colonial authorities saw appropriate food consumption or refusal to
eat as evidence of mental illness. Superintendents in Bombay, like
Victorian asylum doctors, considered food refusal to be 'a symptom or
complication of every psychiatric affliction'.[82] Dr. Maxwell noted how his
patient, Sheik Currim, 'Eats little and seldom with a seeming relish'.
Another patient, who he described as a 'robust Musalman', he noted
'completely refused food'. He diagnosed this patient's case as severe and
restrained him in a straight waistcoat.[83] Food refusal was a valid cause for

---

[78] APR, 1898, p. 9, NLS.

[79] APR, 1876, p. 21, NLS.

[80] APR, 1874, p. 19, NLS.

[81] APR, 1873, p. 45; APR, 1885, p. 7. NLS.

[82] F. Scholz, *Handbook of Mental Science* (Leipzig: Mayer, 1890), p. 32, in Ron Van Deth and Walter Vandereychken, 'Food Refusal and Insanity: Sitophobia and Anorexia Nervosa in Victorian Asylums', *International Journal of Eating Disorders*, Vol. 27, No. 4, May 2000, p. 392.

[83] From Asst. Surgeon J.A. Maxwell to the Chief Secretary to the Government of Bombay, 4 June 1814, GoB, PDD, 1814/368, MSA.

admission into an asylum and asylum staff closely monitored patient appetites as evidence of their mental illness. The colonial notion that mental illness had links to appetite was so staunch that even magistrates sent patients to the asylum simply if they were found fasting. In 1849, Magistrate Bettington sent Brahmin Devram to the insane hospital. He stated:

> Under the influence of religious phrenzy [sic] [the Brahmin] is bent on self-destruction by starvation. Prolonged fasting has added to the mental disturbance ... it is imperative that he be prevented from committing suicide by starvation as if he had taken means to shoot or poison himself ... . He is not judicially cured till he eats food voluntarily. After that as such time as you may consider his bodily health restored he should be sent here with a report as to whether he is a maniac, monomaniac or absolutely free from mental disturbance that further precaution be taken such amount of force as may be necessary to compel him to take nourishment and of precaution and constraint to prevent him destroying himself in any other manner should be resorted to.[84]

Civil Surgeon Gillanders, after observing Devram, disagreed with the Magistrate's opinion about the Brahmin's suicidal tendencies. Once admitted, Devram consumed plantains, sugar, ghee and milk and refused only grains.[85] Surgeon Gillanders concluded that Devram was fasting 'from religious motives' and had no 'intention of committing suicide'.[86] Since food consumption was an indication of the patient's mental health, an integral part of diet treatment involved ensuring that patients had consumed the right quantities of food.

In Bombay's asylums, the staff employed different methods to ensure appropriate consumption of food. Superintendents had a no-toleration policy towards food refusal. They believed that food refusal was more common among Indian patients compared to European patients.[87] Asylum

[84] From the Magistrate of Ahmedabad to the Civil Surgeon, Ahmedabad, 13 August 1849, JD, GoB, GD, 1849/38, MSA.

[85] From the Superintending Surgeon to the Secretary to the Medical Board, 17 August 1849, GoB, GD, 1849/38, MSA.

[86] From the Civil Surgeon to the Magistrate of Ahmedabad, 14 August 1849, GoB, GD, 1849/38, MSA.

[87] APR, 1873–1874, p.17, NLS.

staff commonly resorted to force-feeding patients and even employed patients in restraining other patients who refused food,

> taking the case of patients deliberately set to starving themselves to death. They must be fed. We had a strong young woman here last year – a lady's ayah who took 8 women to hold her while being fed. I do not like to think of the happenings when a stubborn stalwart patient is at the mercy of three unsupervised low class native attendants. Either she is fed or she is brutally treated to make her give in.[88]

Apart from force-feeding, superintendents used the stomach pump to treat patients who refused food. Superintendent Niven at the Colaba Lunatic Asylum described administering food through the stomach pump to a Parsi patient who

> resisted with such determination, that when the beef-tea was administered by means of the stomach pump, as soon as the tube was withdrawn, he ejected the whole of the contents of the stomach.[89]

Superintendents regularly used the stomach pump on patients who 'obstinately'[90] refused food in the asylum, despite the dangers it involved. As Surgeon Gillanders noted: 'Its repeated use is highly dangerous and even in the first application ... had the man, made violent resistance it might have occasioned death'.[91] Apart from the stomach pump, staff also used other methods, such as injecting food through the patient's rectum, as in the case of one Parsi patient, whom asylum staff injected with beef tea in this manner. After all attempts to feed him failed, they discharged the Parsi patient after one month. His relatives reported that within a few days of his return, he began to consume food voluntarily. Superintendent Niven concluded that the willingness of the patient to eat was a sign of his recovery.[92]

---

[88] From Lt. Col. J.P. Barry, Superintendent, Colaba Lunatic Asylum, to the Personal Asst. to the Surgeon General with the Government of Bombay, 11 November 1901, GoB, GD, 1904/57, MSA.

[89] APR, 1873–1874, p. 3, NLS.

[90] APR, 1874–1875, p. 13, NLS.

[91] From the Civil Surgeon, Ahmedabad, to the Magistrate of Ahmedabad, 14 August 1849, GoB, GD, 1849/38, MSA.

[92] APR, 1873–1874, p. 3, NLS.

Doctors interpreted appropriate consumption as a sign of recovery in patients. Sheik Curim, a patient at the Colaba Lunatic Asylum, when admitted in 1814, ate little and 'seldom with seeming relish'. Each month the superintendent recorded his appetite and explained any improvement in appetite as an indication of recovery in his mental health.[93] In 1874, Superintendent Niven reported a case of food refusal of a Parsi who he treated with a stomach pump for two months. Finally, 'one day he was accidentally given a beer, which had the desired effect, as he began to eat soon after on his own accord, and became stout and strong and shows signs of improvement'.[94] Patient appetites were not only monitored but also manipulated. Conformity of Indian patients' appetites to set asylum standards became an indication of their recovery. While setting standards for appropriate consumption, the policy on asylum diet distribution had several contradictions.

Diet distribution reflected pretentious attitudes on the part of asylum authorities. Asylum reports described patient diets as 'liberal', yet 'the greatest economy and supervision' was maintained 'in the regulation and distribution of food'.[95] While superintendents reported the liberality, variety, and generosity of asylum food, they based their assumption of the sufficiency of food for patients, on what they believed patients would have received in their own homes. They claimed that 'the diet of patients leaves nothing to be desired' and that they were 'infinitely better and more liberally fed than their relatives at home'. Furthermore, 'Their diet [was] changed daily, well cooked and properly served'.[96] The Hyderabad Lunatic Asylum only provided two main meals; breakfast at 8 am, dinner at 1.30 pm, and supper at 6–6.30 pm.[97] The sufficiency of the quantity of food was justified by the superintendents by stating that no patients had complained.[98] In order to curtail expenditure, diets were often limited and constrained. For the years 1871–1872, the total expenditure on food for patients in the Presidency was Rs. 40,993; in the following year, the

[93] From Asst. Surgeon J.A. Maxwell to the Chief Secretary to the Government of Bombay, 4 June 1814, GoB, PDD, 1814/368, MSA.

[94] APR, 1874–1975 p. 13, NLS.

[95] APR, 1874–1875, p. 11, NLS.

[96] From the Superintendent of the Poona Asylum to the Personal Asst. to the Surgeon General with the Government of Bombay, GoB, GD, 1905/55, MSA.

[97] Rules for the Lunatic Asylums in the Bombay Presidency (Up to 1907), GoB, GD, 1908/80, MSA.

[98] APR, 1873–1874, p. 44, NLS.

amount reduced to Rs. 29,073, and by 1873–1874 the dietary charges for the asylums of the Presidency stood at Rs. 20,613. The Presidency asylums made a saving of Rs. 19,695 in a short span of three years, 'not withstanding an increase in the number of lunatics'.[99]

Apart from solid food, drinks played an important role in manipulation, control, and in the creation of distinctions between patients. Milk was the most commonly administered drink. Superintendents used milk, curd, or buttermilk to induce Indian patients to work.[100] There was also a special 'Milk Diet' for some patients, consisting of milk, rice, and sugar.[101] Superintendents reserved alcoholic drinks for Europeans and those whom they considered to be Europeanized. They gave beer and wine to Europeans and occasionally to Eurasians. Asylum staff indulged mixed race people with a European diet because they deemed it 'beneficial to their health'.[102] They also occasionally gave Parsi patients a beer, as in the case of Dr. Niven's patient who was 'accidentally given a beer'.[103] Only the Colaba Lunatic Asylum supplied tea for patients.[104] Superintendents used tea to distinguish Indian patients who were European in their habits and customs. The Superintendent at Colaba reported that at his asylum, Christians and Parsis were given tea because they were 'very fond of tea and it would amount to an act of cruelty to deprive them of that article of diet'.[105] At times, asylum staff gave other local drinks to Indian patients. It was unlikely that the superintendent was aware of this practice, since it occurred at night when the superintendent was not at the asylum. Sajan Curim, a former patient, elucidated that the night asylum staff locked him up in the asylum and gave him 'a small cup of *fenny*' (a local alcoholic drink brewed from cashew). The ward boys, however, refused to give him water to dilute the alcohol. The Superintendent at the Colaba Lunatic Asylum became aware of the same only when Curim wrote a letter of complaint to him regarding the behaviour of the ward boys.[106] Like solid food,

[99] APR, 1873–1874, pp. 7–8, NLS.

[100] APR, 1876, p. 27, NLS.

[101] Rules of the Bombay Lunatic Asylum, 1864, GoB, GD, 1862–1864/15, MSA.

[102] APR, 1873–1874, p. 7, NLS.

[103] APR, 1874–1875 p.13, NLS.

[104] Asylum General Rules (Bombay Presidency) submitted with Letter 1103 from the Surgeon General, Indian Medical Department, 13 April 1874, GD, 1874/32, MSA.

[105] APR, 1873–1874, p. 8, NLS.

[106] From Sajan Curim to the Superintendent, Lunatic Asylum Colaba, 17 October 1891, GoB, GD, 1893/75, MSA.

asylum staff regulated the quality and quantity of drink to exert control over patients.

The superintendents also set boundaries[107] for negotiations in diet treatment. They permitted hybridity only in food preparation, while they maintained strict control over other stages of diet treatment. Although colonial agencies allowed Indian food and spices and even separate cooks[108] in the asylum, they determined the quantity and quality of diet. At the asylum, they permitted those practices that reinforced ideas of rigidity of caste and religion. The colonial government even went to the extent of prescribing specific ingredients and their quantities in the Rules of the Bombay Lunatic Asylum. The Native Diet Scale of 1864 listed the recipe for the curry paste for use in Bombay's asylums. Superintendents had to 'inspect and approve' the 'daily supply of every description of articles of diet'.[109] 'Patients who refuse[d] food or whose appetite is poor' had 'to be regularly reported to the superintendent since such cases called for individual attention'.[110] The asylum apportioned patient diets according to colonial prerequisites, indicating a subjective liberality on the part of medical authorities.

Asylum staff manipulated patients' bodies through food so that they were strong enough for work but weak enough for control. Doctors believed that Indian patients were physically weaker, since they were 'debilitated through prior want and exposure'.[111] However, the amount they spent on them for diet was far less than what they spent on European or Eurasian diets. Annual yearly costs of patient diets prove the maintenance of racial disparities and discrimination towards Indian patients. While the annual average expenditure on a European patient at Colaba was 200Rs. 9a.1p, that for Parsis and Jews was 114Rs. 0a. 2p. and the cost for dieting Hindus and Muslims was 64Rs. 6a. 2p.. The average annual cost of patient diets in the 'native' asylums of the Presidency was less than half of the average cost for diets for Europeans. At Poona, the average yearly cost of diet for an Indian patient was merely 65Rs. 11a. 5p.; at Dharwar it stood at 41Rs. 14a. 3p.; at Ahmedabad it amounted to 56Rs.

---

[107] Nandy, *The Intimate Enemy*, p. 3.

[108] The Naupada Asylum appointed a Brahmin cook in 1911. Statement of Accounts for the Bai Putlibai Trust, GoB, GD, 1911/117, MSA.

[109] Rules of the Bombay Lunatic Asylum, 1864, GoB, GD, 1862–1864/15, MSA.

[110] Rules for the Lunatic Asylums in the Bombay Presidency (Up to 1907), GoB, GD, 1908/80, MSA.

[111] A.H.L. Fraser and C.J.H. Warden, Notes on Asylum Administration, 7 August 1894, GoB, GD, 1895/77, MSA.

5a. 7p.; and Hyderabad had the lowest dietary cost of 34Rs. 5a and 8.p. The stark differences in diet scales shows the importance of economic logic, where those who laboured did not reap equal benefits. Indian patients laboured to maintain the asylum, but they received meagre amounts of food. Ironically, asylum agencies provided sumptuous meals to European and Eurasian patients, but they refused to employ them on the pretext that the asylums lacked suitable work for them.[112]

Diet treatment shared a close relationship with chemical treatment of patients; in some instances, it even replaced chemical treatment. Dr. Maxwell noted how 'vegetable acids and bark along with a nourishing diet and occasional laxatives were administered as treatment'. Chemical treatment of the body included the use of mild aperients, cold affusions, aertake or muriate of morphia.[113] Medicine served in 'regulating bowels' and as sedatives. Doctors used 'Potassium bromadium, belladonna, conium, Indian hemp and morphia' to 'quiet excitement and induce sleep'.[114] However, medicine (drugs) held a 'useful but subordinate position' in the treatment of patients.[115] Doctors believed that a 'good hearty meal and a stimulant' was the 'best sedative' and therefore, they treated patients by giving them 'plenty of food'.[116] Food, when it replaced medicine served the purpose of keeping patients alert for work.[117] Superintendents mostly administered drugs to new patients.[118] A patient at the Colaba Lunatic Asylum complained to the government of this practice, stating that 'medicine is not properly given; whatever is indispensable it is never given'.[119] The use of medicine was limited because of financial constraints. Even the most important of drugs like hyoscyamine was struck out of the list of necessities for the new asylum at Naupada to make the budget more economical. As the Superintendent at Colaba noted, 'Economic torpidity paralyzed all efforts' towards effective medical treatment.[120]

---

[112] APR, 1898, p. 9, NLS.

[113] Annual Report of the Bombay Lunatic Asylum, 31 March 1849, Board Collections, 1849–1851 (1851–1852), F42450, IOR, BL, London.

[114] APR, 1874–1875, p. 9, NLS.

[115] APR, 1873–1874, p. 17, NLS.

[116] APR, 1873–1874, p. 4, NLS.

[117] APR, 1874–1874, p. 44, NLS.

[118] APR, 1873–1874, p. 44, NLS.

[119] From Sajan Curim (former patient) through the Surgeon General to the Secretary to Government, 16 October 1893, GoB, GD, 1893/75, MSA.

[120] From Lt. Col. Barry, Superintendent, Colaba Lunatic Asylum, to the Personal Asst. to the Surgeon General with the Government of Bombay, 25 June 1904, GoB, GD, 1907/81, MSA.

THE 'COMMON-SENSE' TREATMENT OF INDIAN INSANITY

Asylum foodscapes facilitated the 'creation and recreation' of social distinctions and regulations.[121] Food as material culture became a means to 'produce and reinforce' both race and caste.[122] The foodscape of the asylum was a place of 'historical encounters', where caste was colonially constructed. Such a construction often erased the heterogeneous character of Indian society.[123] The superintendents projected caste as a basis for food refusal among all Indian patients. Occasionally, the superintendent or assistant surgeon in charge would permit patients to practice 'caste prejudices' around food.[124] In 1911, a separate Brahmin cook was appointed using funding from the Bai Putlibai Trust,[125] which was originally set up to supplement 'the diet, clothing and medical comforts provided ... for high class[caste] Hindu and other inmates of the asylum'.[126] Racial distinctions were harder to maintain in the asylum. Spatial constraints in Bombay's asylums limited the classification of patients and erased boundaries between European, Eurasian, and Indian patients.[127] So, maintaining different diet scales based on race was essential to 'producing and reinforcing'[128] ideas of racial superiority that staff failed to maintain through spatial segregation.[129] Asylum foodscapes represented colonial cultural attitudes towards food in its colonies, in which it remained a space for articulating 'social distance' and separation.[130] Superintendents made exceptions in diet for mixed race patients or Parsis who they perceived as 'quite Europeanized in regard to social and personal habits of life'.[131]

Hybridity in diet treatment practices existed only to a certain extent, and it added to the ambiguous nature of treatment practices. David Arnold

[121] Rachel Slocum, 'Race in the Study of Food', *Progress in Human Geography*, Vol. 35, No. 3, 2011, p. 315.

[122] Ibid., p. 313.

[123] Nicholas Dirks, *Castes of Mind: Colonialism and the Making of Modern India* (Princeton: Princeton University Press, 2001), p. 5.

[124] From the Superintendent of the Lunatic Asylum, Colaba, to the Secretary to the Inspector General, Medical Department, GoB, GD, 1862–1864/15, MSA.

[125] Statement of Accounts for the Bai Putlibai Trust, GoB, GD, 1911/117, MSA.

[126] PWD, No. 98-C.W.366, 25 February 1891, GoB, GD, 1901/66, MSA.

[127] Extracts from the Reports of Visitors of the Lunatic Asylum, Colaba, 19 January 1869, GoB, GD, 1869/4, MSA.

[128] Slocum, 'Race in the Study of Food', p. 313.

[129] APR, 1873–1874, pp. 7–8, NLS.

[130] Cecelia Leong-Salobir, *Food Culture in Colonial Asia: A Taste of Empire* (London and New York: Routledge, 2011), p. 8.

[131] APR, 1873–1874, pp. 7–8, NLS.

argued that the colonial acceptance of hybridity in western medicine was a means of gaining the acceptance of local communities.[132] Hybridity in diet practices performed a similar function. While it helped maintain racial separateness, asylum staff adopted it to make the asylum more relevant to Indian people. Hybrid diet practices, however, also set the 'psychological limits' within which Indian patients could express their self-consciousness. These 'limits' are evident in the control and prescription of the quantity and quality of food for Indian patients.[133] Asylum staff strictly maintained these limits at different stages of food production, preparation, consumption, and distribution. Moreover, asylum staff set predetermined boundaries on the extent to which patients could negotiate their diet. They permitted only those negotiations that facilitated the creation and reinforcement of colonial stereotypes in the diet treatment process.

The asylum foodscape represented a space of control and contradiction. The display of compassion towards Indian sensibilities, by permitting hybridity, contrasted with the discrimination in quantities of food provided for Indian patients. Asylum reports projected asylum foodscapes as one in which patients were always well fed. Appropriate feeding, however, often meant meagrely fed and force-fed. While asylum staff permitted Indian food, they meticulously prescribed quantities of food. The asylum foodscape represented the 'messy, mixed up and interconnected nature'[134] of colonial-local encounters.

OCCUPATIONAL THERAPY

In Bombay's asylums, occupation as a form of treatment gained increasing significance in the latter half of the nineteenth century. Superintendent Campbell reported to the government that the Colaba Lunatic Asylum had no proper facilities for occupation prior to 1850.[135] Even though the government made additions to the asylum in the mid-nineteenth century, until 1869 there was 'no space for recreation, amusement or employment'.[136]

[132] Arnold, *Colonizing the Body*, p. 251.

[133] Nandy, *The Intimate Enemy*, p. 3.

[134] Ian Cook and Michelle Harrison, 'Cross Over Food: Rematerializing Postcolonial Geographies', *Transactions of the Institute of British Geographers*, No. 28, 2003, p. 310.

[135] Report on the Lunatic Asylum at Colaba for the Year Ending 1852, GoB, GD, 1853/48, MSA.

[136] From the Inspector General, IMD, to the Adjunct General of the Army, 12 January 1869, GoB, GD, 1869/4, MSA.

During this time, clothing and diet as treatment continued to remain significant, since it prepared the Indian body for work. By the latter half of that century, capitalist ideals increasingly affected the public health care system in the colony. Economic viability and profitability became the criteria for assessing the success of health care institutions. This assessment, in turn, influenced treatment methods within the colonial asylums.

The colonial government in asylum treatment practices reinforced capitalist principles. Over the course of the nineteenth century, the Indian landscape changed from an ambiguous political entity into a 'regulated empire'.[137] With increasing regulation, the state ordered the colony through its institutionalization. The lunatic asylum as once such institution helped the ordering of the empire by 'mobilizing labour'.[138] Colonial agencies envisioned the transformation of the asylum not only into a self-sufficient colonial enterprise but also into a profitable one. The Annual Asylum Report of the Presidency in 1849 contained the first table classifying previous occupations of patients.[139] The classification of patients based on occupation was a means to mobilize 'profitable labour'. Labour could then be extracted 'from pliable inmates who [had] learnt some trade'.[140]

This section argues that the purpose of labouring patients was not merely to maintain the 'asylum efficiency logic',[141] but rather to maximize profits. The colonial state reinforced occupation as moral therapy, not because of its popularity as a Victorian treatment method or as light work that would 'produce a salutary effect over their disease minds',[142] but because patient labour would produce and maximize profits. Colonial authorities pressurized asylum doctors to compromise on treatment for the sake of profits. Bombay's asylum superintendents faced a peculiar problem in this matter. Local conditions forced them to modify moral

---

[137] Ranajit Guha, *Dominance Without Hegemony: History and Power in Colonial India* (Cambridge, London: Harvard University Press, 1997), pp. 25, 27.

[138] Ibid., p. 27.

[139] Annual Report of the Bombay Lunatic Asylum, 31 March 1849, Board Collections, 1849–1851 (1851–1852), F42450, IOR, BL.

[140] W.J. Moore Esq., Surgeon General with the Government of Bombay, to the Secretary to the Government of Bombay, General Department, Bombay, 7 October 1885, Home Department, GoI, Medical Proceedings, November, Nos. 21 and 22, NAI, New Delhi.

[141] Roman et al., 'No Time for Nostalgia!: Asylum-making, Medicalized Colonialism in British Columbia (1859–97) and Artistic Praxis for Social Transformation', *International Journal of Qualitative Studies in Education*, Vol. 22, No. 1, 2009, p. 34.

[142] From the Civil Surgeon, Dharwar, to Officer Simon Esquire, 3 August 1844, GoB, GD, 1844/34-840, MSA.

therapy. Hybridized to suit the ground realities of each asylum, moral management of the patients through occupation failed to produce expected profits in Bombay. The asylums in Bombay lagged in profit making when compared to the asylums in the other parts of colonial India.[143]

Bombay's asylum superintendents faced several hindrances in getting their patients occupied profitably. The Superintendent of the Colaba Lunatic Asylum complained: 'There is much difficulty in finding employment for the lunatics particularly in reference to remunerative industry'.[144] Superintendents bemoaned the interference of 'religious superstitions and caste [that] were obstructing their patients from working'.[145] Moreover, superintendents reported that it was rare to find 'skilled workmen of any kind in the asylums of this country, at all events in this presidency'.[146] Physical conditions of patients also obstructed their participation in remunerative labour. The Superintendent at Dharwar noted that most patients were paupers and were 'mentally and physically the lowest of the low'. Superintendents also reported that the patients were too weak to work because relatives brought them in when they were in the final stages of a disease.[147] Superintendents also lamented: 'A large number of their patients … [were] unfit for steady or profitable labour'.[148] Apart from the condition and preferences of patients, local conditions also limited the superintendents' options for suitable employment for patients.

Spatial limitations, water shortages, and weather and soil conditions limited the superintendents' choice of remunerative occupations for patients.[149] At the Colaba and Poona Lunatic Asylums, 'Outdoor or field labour which … [was] considered one of the best means of cure … [was] utterly unimaginable in the asylum' and 'the means of employing lunatics … [were] extremely limited'.[150] Both these asylums had no space for

[143] From the Offg. Secretary to the Government of India to Secretary to the Government of Bombay, 13 August 1894, GoI, Home Department, P 4554, IOR, BL.

[144] APR, 1873–1874, p. 11, NLS.

[145] Asst. Surgeon Lunatic Asylum, Colaba, to the Secretary of the Medical Board, 21 February 1847, GoB, GD, 1847/41, MSA.

[146] APR, 1873–1874, p. 22, NLS.

[147] Asst. Surgeon, Lunatic Asylum, Colaba, to the Secretary of the Medical Board, 21 February 1847, GoB, GD, 1847/41, MSA.

[148] APR, 1899, p. 12, NLS.

[149] APR, 1873–1874, pp. 10–11, 22, NLS.

[150] In Poona, as a memo stated: 'Outdoor occupation, so largely conducive to the amelioration of the patient [was] largely wanting'. Memorandum of the Final Proceeding of the Visitors of the Lunatic Asylum, Poona, GoB, GD, 1871/34, MSA; APR, 1873–1874, pp. 21–24, NLS.

undertaking dairy farming or major agricultural work. The asylums were also located in central parts of the town where land was expensive to buy. The Surgeon General noted that even at the asylums at Ahmedabad and Ratnagiri local conditions were unfavourable for starting dairy farms for the employment of patients since there was 'no sufficient demand for dairy produce'.[151] Furthermore, agriculture or gardening enterprises were largely unsuccessful because of water shortage. At Colaba, Superintendent Niven explained that except during the monsoon, the water supply was 'deficient at all times'.[152] There was barely enough water for domestic purposes and 'none to sluice the drains' or for gardening.[153] Agricultural labour or gardening, which was considered the 'best suitable' employment for 'wandering beggars and religious mendicants', was 'impracticable for want of soil and water'.[154] The Cowasji Jehangir Lunatic Asylum, Hyderabad, had no spatial limitations. Patients grew grape and mango crops, but the produce was 'scanty' because of inadequate rainfall.[155] Local conditions affected the prospect of profits from Bombay's lunatic asylums.

With an increasing focus on profitability in the latter half of the nineteenth century, the colonial state tried to seek a solution to the lack of profitability in Bombay's asylums. While superintendents in Bombay wanted to focus on gardening and cultivation to employ patients,[156] the government did not consider this very remunerative.[157] Dr. R.G. Lord, the Acting Civil Surgeon at Poona, still encouraged it since it would ensure a regular supply of 'food and vegetables for the European population'.[158] The government considered manufactures like 'oil pressing, dairy and farming' most profitable. Surgeon General P.S. Turnbill, in his report on the lack of profitability in asylums in the Presidency, discussed possibilities of employing patients not just to keep them

---

[151] From the Surgeon General with the Government of Bombay to the Secretary to the Government of Bombay, 15 February 1893, GOB, GD, 1893/68, MSA.

[152] APR, 1873–1874, p. 1, NLS.

[153] APR, 1873–1874, p. 11, NLS.

[154] APR, 1874–1874, p. 11, NLS.

[155] APR, 1876, p. 25, NLS.

[156] Proceedings of the Government of Bombay, General Department, No. 2056, 3 Nov 1868, Home Department, Public Proceedings, 1869, GOI, OC 218/97, NAI.

[157] APR, 1886, p. 1, NLS.

[158] From Dr. R. Lord, Acting Civil Surgeon, Poona, to the Deputy Inspector General of Hospitals, 23 June 1864, GoB, GD, 1862–1864/15, MSA.

occupied or productive, but rather in occupations that would maximize profits:

> I beg to state that the results of the manufacturing operations must continue to compare unfavourably with those of other provinces so long as the facilities and circumstances remain as they are. In the Colaba Asylum, for instance space is so limited that agricultural operations are impossible and industries such as oil pressing, dairy, farming, &c, from which large profits are said to be made elsewhere cannot be profitably carried out. To put our asylums on par with asylums in other parts of India really good arable land in the vicinity of the asylum with a good supply of water for agricultural purposes will be necessary and plant and machinery of a good and modern description for manufacturing purposes will be required. At Ahmedabad and Poona, perhaps even at Hyderabad, the conditions are more favourable than elsewhere but land and machinery are required and I am not even sure if supplied the results will commensurate with the outlay. So far as I have been able to judge from cursory inspections, I do not think the soil in Naupada will in anyway compare with that of Bengal and the North-western Provinces, and the results must always be unfavourable from an agricultural and financial point of view.[159]

The memorandum of the government in response to the Hemp Commission also reiterated that 'employment of insanes in gardens and fields be restricted to what is probably absolutely necessary'. Instead, it recommended that superintendents employ their patients in 'construction of buildings, as domestic servants and in dairy farming'.[160]

The colonial government justified its proposal to use patient labour in manufactures rather than in gardening or agriculture by claiming that agriculture was perilous to the health of patients. Dr. Rice, Surgeon General with the Government of India, in his reply to the members of the Hemp Commission recommended against Indian patients' employment in agriculture, since it was harmful for them. Instead, he recommended employing patients in manufacturing, since 'lunatics employed on manufactures soon become quiet and manageable; they would go on for hours in their work apparently contented and easy in their

---

[159] APR, 1894, pp. 116–118, NLS.

[160] Administration of Lunatic Asylums in India, Home Department Notes from the Government of Bengal, No. 3680, 25 August 1896, Simla Records 4, Medical Proceedings, August 1896, No. 188-232, NAI.

minds'.[161] At the close of the century, the state placed an increasing emphasis on manufacturing rather than on farming or gardening because of the higher yield of profits. For the Bombay Presidency, the government specifically endorsed the establishment of dairy farms attached to its lunatic asylums.

The government initiated a discussion for starting such dairy farms in 1892. The Surgeon General of Bombay, in reply to a government proposal, had reported that dairy farms in lunatic asylums were impracticable and unprofitable because of spatial limitations and the lack of a market for dairy produce.[162] The government, however, overrode the Surgeon General's conclusions and appointed the Survey Commissioner to assess the availability of land adjacent to the asylums.[163] The Survey Commissioner concluded that only the Dharwar Asylum was viable for establishing a dairy farm. The farm, he explained, would be 'financially remunerative' and would ensure a steady supply of dairy products to the jail, civil, and military hospitals.[164] In 1893, the Surgeon General staunchly objected the establishment of dairy farms. He sternly remarked:

> I do not think that a Lunatic asylum is a place for a commercial undertaking of any kind, much less that of dairy farming, which requires so much nicety of manipulation and skilled attention ...[165]

The government finally abandoned the plan of dairy farming; however, profitability remained the main concern of the colonial state in maintaining lunatic asylums.

At times even asylum staff prioritized profitability over the care and treatment of patients. The Superintendent at Hyderabad noted how he avoided giving drugs to patients to keep them alert for work. Instead, he

[161] Dr. Rice, Surgeon General, Further Notes on the Remarks by Messrs. Fraser and Warden on the Management of Lunatic Asylums in India, 24 October 1894, Home Department, GoI, Simla Records, Medical Proceedings, March 1895, No. 97-99, NAI.
[162] From the Surgeon General with the Government of Bombay to the Secretary to the Government, 15 February 1893, GOB, GD, 1893/68, MSA.
[163] From the Survey Commissioner and Director, Land Records and Agriculture, to the Chief Secretary to the Government of Bombay, 17 June 1893, GoB, GD, 1893/68, MSA.
[164] From the Survey Commissioner and Director, Land Records and Agriculture, to the Chief Secretary to the Government of Bombay, 17 June 1893, GoB, GD, 1893/68, MSA.
[165] From the Surgeon General with the Government of Bombay to the Secretary to the Government of Bombay, 27 July 1893, GoB, GD, 1893/68, MSA.

used 'curd, tobacco and snuff to induce them to work'.[166] The asylum at Hyderabad, completed in 1871[167] and built with a donation of Rs. 50,000 from Cowasji Jehangir,[168] a Parsi businessman, also provides evidence of prioritization of profits over treatment. Despite the huge donation, the government chose an unhealthy location close to the river Indus[169] for the asylum in order to obtain water for crops. In 1885, the asylum was merely a large enclosure with two to three acres of cultivable land and sheds with platforms for patients to sleep.[170] In 1875, while the superintendent reported that the health of patients was extremely poor because of the previous year's flooding, he made the patients labour along with prisoners to build a boundary wall for the asylum.[171] In 1906, the *Bombay Samachar* criticizing the Triennial Asylum Report of the Presidency for the years 1903–1905, reported that patients who were 'past the hope of recovery were discharged and made over to their relatives or guardians'.[172] Patients who were beyond recovery were non-profitable, and doctors therefore discharged them to their families or relatives.

Unable to reach goals of profit and facing pressure from the colonial government, Bombay's superintendents responded by offering patient labour to other institutions. This outsourcing of patient labour was a manifestation of hybridity in treatment practices. Superintendents tailored occupation as a means of moral therapy to suit local conditions. Apart from domestic work, superintendents employed patients in 'extra-mural work'.[173] They made patients carry provisions or water to the asylum or they sent them to work in nearby institutions as cleaners and gardeners. Asylum staff also used patients to serve the needs of the PWD for manual jobs like cutting trees, which was not particularly appropriate as work for mentally unstable patients.[174] It therefore seems that occupational therapy was not just about teaching patients the values of order and discipline; it

---

[166] APR, 1873–1874, p. 44, NLS.
[167] From the Commissioner in Sindh to the Governor and President in Council, 11 July 1871, Kurachee, GoB, GD, 1871/ 34, MSA.
[168] A.W. Hughes, *A Gazetteer of the Province of Sindh* (London: George Bell and Sons, 1874), p. 206.
[169] APR, 1875, p. 24, NLS.
[170] APR, 1885, p. 7, NLS.
[171] APR, 1875, p. 25, NLS.
[172] RNP, *Bombay Samachar*, 5 June 1906, 1906, J–J, GoB, MSA.
[173] APR, 1898, p. 9, NLS.
[174] APR, 1896, p. 7; APR, 1897, p. 25, NLS.

also served as a means to deploy them in the service of the Empire. Bombay's asylums became a source of *begar* labour (unpaid forced labour) for public works.[175] While superintendents lent out patients to labour in other government departments or nearby institutions, local communities objected to the practice. Local communities complained that the practice was harmful since it could lead to freak accidents.[176]

Occupational therapy, hybridized to create new forms of labour, was far more exploitative. The definitions as to what constituted light labour (for exercise and therapy) and hard labour were often unclear. Occupational therapy ranged from gardening to the use of patient labour to maintain other public institutions. In Poona, patients were 'employed from time to time at the Collectors *Kutcherry* (office) and the Sassoon hospital'.[177] Female patients ground grain not only for the asylum, but also for outside dealers in the city who had contracts with the asylum.[178] Women at the asylum in Ahmedabad ground grain for the Huttesing Hospital.[179] At Hyderabad, the Superintendent made patients provide free labour for the PWD, saving it Rs. 2000 in expenses.[180] At Colaba, patients paved the 'lanes and corners of the ground', 'laid dry rubble stone pitching for the warders' *chawl*,[181] and painted articles of the asylum like bathing tubs.[182]

---

[175] Ranajit Guha argued that the colonial state used indigenous people for *begar* or forced labour for public works, for ordering the Empire. The policy of forced labour was mostly used on poorer classes like the *paharis* and *adivasis*. They had to provide various labour services for colonial officials, ranging from carrying baggage to constructing roads for 'no remuneration at all'. See Guha, *Dominance without Hegemony*, p. 26.

[176] The *Akbari Saudagar* in 1871 criticized asylum authorities for making patients carry provisions from the commissariat stores to the asylum during the sultry hours of the day. RNP, *Akbari Sowdagar*, 13 April 1871, K 406, J–D, PG. 1-543, GoB, MSA.

[177] APR, 1876, p. 18; From the Superintendent, Lunatic Asylum, Poona, to the Surgeon General with the Government of Bombay, 20 January 1911, GoB, GD, 1911/ 117, MSA; From the Superintendent, Central Lunatic Asylum, Yerawada, Poona, to the Personal Asst. to the Surgeon General, GoB, GD, 1915/697, MSA.

[178] APR, 1876, p. 18, NLS.

[179] APR, 1876, p. 21, NLS; Similar practices of employing patients were also used in asylums around the world. See Geoffery Reaume, 'Insane Asylum Inmates' Labour in Ontario, 1841–1900', in James Moran and David Wright (eds.), *Mental Health and Canadian Society* (Montreal & Kingston, London, Ithaca: McGill-Queen's University Press, 2006), pp. 69–96; Sally Swartz, 'The Black Insane in Cape, 1891–1920', *Journal of Southern African Studies*, Vol. 21, No. 3, September 1995, pp. 411–414.

[180] APR, 1876, p. 27, NLS.

[181] *Chawl* is a type of housing unit in India used by the lower-middle or poor classes.

[182] APR, 1873–1874, p. 6, NLS.

The Colaba Lunatic Asylum also employed patients for carrying sand or mud from the foreshore for the garden or for reclamation purposes.[183] One superintendent noted that patients were '…employed as supplementary servants an estimate value of which has not been taken into account'.[184] For a large number of patients, doctors could not ascertain their previous occupation.[185] This class of patients provided a labour pool that the asylum could retrain in skills that would maximize its profits. By 1906, Bombay's asylums had factories attached to them, and by 1911 asylum agencies trained patients in specific skills to employ them in those factories. Factory work mainly included weaving and manufacturing cloth.[186] In 1913, through manufactures, Bombay's asylums had managed to make a profit of Rs. 5189 0a 11p.[187]

The hybridity of occupational therapy limited the profitability of the asylums. Surgeon General James Cleghorn tried to justify this to asylum medical staff by reiterating: "The results financially are not a success but the object in introducing manufactures and other forms of labour in the asylum was not to show profit'.[188] The government, nevertheless, was very clear about its vision for the asylum and criticized Bombay's superintendents:

> In reviewing the returns of last year, the governor general in council remarked that the arrangements regarding manufacture in lunatic asylums in the Bombay Presidency appeared to be in a very backward condition, and a statement was given showing that they compared unfavourably with the returns of most provinces in India. The Government of India regret to observe nevertheless, that very little improvement took place during the year under review. In the asylum at Colaba which has by far the largest number of lunatics in the Bombay Presidency, only 32 per cent of the inmates

[183] APR, 1873–1874, p. 4, NLS.

[184] APR, 1898, p. 9, NLS.

[185] APR, 1915, p. 2, NLS.

[186] Report on the Lunatic Asylums under the Government of Bombay, Triennial, 1906–1908, p. 5; Report on the Lunatic Asylums for the Government of Bombay, Triennial, 1909–1911, p. 6, NLS

[187] Triennial Report of the Lunatic Asylums under the Government of Bombay, 1912–1914, p. 30, NLS.

[188] Note by the Director-General, Indian Medical Service, on the Reports Lunatic Asylums, Under Local Governments and Administrations for the Year 1895, Home Department, Medical Proceedings, Simla Records, September 1896, Nos. 65-90, NAI.

were employed on manufactures ... the rate of profits ... is far below that show in any other Province.[189]

Profitability became the index to measure the success of the colonial asylum. Bombay's meagre profits proved its failure as a colonial enterprise. The beginning of World War I in 1914 brought in a steady flow of patients[190] who were profitable for labour. These patients mobilized for labour brought financial stability, profits, and respite to an ailing asylum system. In 1914, Bombay's Asylums had incurred a loss of Rs 207 4a 1p and had a credit of profit of Rs 5189. Two years into the war, however, asylum financial records showed no loss and a profit of Rs 8130 1a 7p from manufactures.[191]

Conclusion

The 'common-sense' treatment of insanity that primarily entailed clothing, feeding, and occupying patients remained the chief method of treating Indian patients. Clothing treatment was rooted in the ideology of the civilizing mission. Superintendents lived the 'fantasy of the civilizing mission'[192] by properly clothing the violent Indian male and promiscuous Indian female patients. The colonial bid to clothe the 'native' appropriately through the adoption of uniform attire was culturally insensitive, since it failed to take into consideration cultural modalities of Indian clothing. Colonial attempts at clothing Indian patients were fundamentally a 'cultural project of control'.[193] Such colonial efforts to control the Indian body are also evident in the asylum foodscape. Asylum staff assigned Indian patients with tasks of preparing and producing their own food, while consumption and distribution of food were strictly controlled. The inequality in food distribution represented the influence of capitalist ideals, as Indian patients had to labour in the production and preparation of their food; however, their diet quantities remained meagre compared to

---

[189] From the Offg. Secretary to the Government of India to Secretary to the Government of Bombay, 13 August 1894, GoI, Home Department, P 4554, IOR, BL.

[190] From the Surgeon General to the Government of Bombay, 3 August 1935, GoB, GD, 4192IVB:81, MSA, in James Mills, 'Modern Psychiatry in India, 1858–1947', *History of Psychiatry*, Vol. 12, No. 431, 2001, pp. 446–447.

[191] APR, 1916, p. 26, NLS.

[192] Mills, '"More Important to Civilize than Subdue"', pp. 171–190.

[193] Cohn, *Colonialism and its Forms of Knowledge*, p. xi.

European patients. Diet treatment prepared the Indian body for labour. Occupation became increasingly significant as a form of treatment in the latter half of the nineteenth century. The chief goal of the colonial state in propagating occupation therapy was to maximize profitability and mobilize labour to serve the empire rather than to encourage non-restraint or moral therapy.

The adoption of hybrid clothing, diet, and occupation treatments facilitated the continuation of the asylum system. Asylum staff permitted such hybrid treatment practices since it served as a means to control Indian expressions of resistance. By permitting hybridity, superintendents set the 'psychological limits'[194] for such expressions. On one hand, hybridity in treatment practices enabled the subversion of Indian sensibilities; on the other hand, it undermined the hegemony of the colonial state. The hybrid nature of occupational therapy reduced profitability and made the asylum a liability to the government. Hybridity reduced profits, but it did not reduce the degree of control or the extent of abuse of the patients.

The asylum failed as a colonial medical institution in Bombay because superintendents preferred treating Indian insanity in a 'common-sense' way—using clothing, diet, and labour as treatment. James Mills has argued that 'modern' psychiatric practices were implemented in Indian asylums from 1858 to 1947.[195] Mills' argument can be applied to the Indian Mental Hospital at Ranchi that made considerable progress in implementing principles and treatment based on modern psychiatry by 1930. At the Ranchi Mental Hospital, Superintendent Dhunjibhoy began using treatment methods like hydrotherapy and psychoanalysis on Indian patients.[196] Nevertheless, he continued the practice of occupational therapy 'as vigorously as before'.[197] In contrast to the Ranchi hospital, Bombay's lunatic asylums did not implement modern methods of psychi-

[194] Nandy, *The Intimate Enemy*, p. 3.

[195] James Mills, 'The History of Modern Psychiatry in India, 1858–1947', *History of Psychiatry*, Vol. 12, 2001, pp. 434–435.

[196] Waltraud Ernst, *Colonialism and Transnational Psychiatry: The Development of an Indian Mental Hospital in British India, 1925–1930* (London, New York: Anthem Press, 2013), pp. 178–194. While the Indian Mental Hospital at Ranchi reached its zenith under the superintendence of Dr. Dhunjibhoy, its condition deteriorated after India's independence. See Waltraud Ernst, 'The Indianization of Colonial Medicine: The Case of Psychiatry in Early-Twentieth-Century British India', *NTM International Journal of History &Ethics of Natural Sciences, Technology and Medicine*, Vol. 20, May 2012, p. 71.

[197] Annual Report on the Working of the Ranchi Indian Mental Hospital, Kanke in Bihar and Orissa for the Year 1930, p. 9, NLS.

atric treatment. Occupational therapy and diet remained the chief methods of treating Indian insanity. Even in 1927, Bombay's superintendents continued to complain of the 'poor facilities' for occupational therapy.[198] In 1933, the Annual Asylum Report for the Presidency noted the employment of patients in 'gardening, weaving, bidi-making, tailoring, sewing, carpentry and cane work' and other domestic duties.[199] Bombay's lunatic asylums were essentially custodial, providing 'too much treatment and too little care'.[200]

The lack of 'care' is also apparent from the asylum soundscapes. The next chapter, then, examines the colonial asylum soundscape as evidence for the lack of the implementation of modern treatment. Noise was a common feature of asylum soundscapes around the world; however, the lack of regulation of sound was a distinct feature of asylums in Bombay. The chapter uses the asylum soundscape as evidence for the failure of the asylum as a colonial medical institution.

[198] Annual Report on the Mental Hospitals in the Bombay Presidency for the Year (AR) 1926, p. 7, NLS.

[199] AR, 1933, p. 3, NLS.

[200] Dr. Niven, Superintendent of the Colaba Lunatic Asylum, noted that while the Lunacy Acts made provisions for the 'care and treatment' of patients in lunatic asylums, most often 'poor lunatics' received 'too much treatment and too little care'. APR, 1873–1874, p. 21, NLS.

CHAPTER 5

Unsound Soundscapes: Shrieks, Shouts, and Songs

The tiny island of Colaba, with its ideal view of the Bombay harbour and the surrounding countryside, was an island of paradoxes. A 'noisy' village covered a part of the island, while two burial grounds (English and Muslim) covered the other. On its western shore lay the Colaba Lunatic Asylum. The location of the asylum afforded pleasant winds from every direction, except the East. The upper storeys of the building commanded 'picturesque and pleasing views'.[1] The pleasant views from the Colaba Lunatic Asylum, however, contrasted with the sounds emanating from it. John Murray, in his account of Bombay city, observed that the English cemetery, though 'tolerably well kept, [was] rendered dismal by having a lunatic asylum adjoining it ... and walking about to examine the tombs the cries of the unhappy inmates are constantly heard'.[2]

The soundscape of the colonial asylum was an extremely noisy one. Noise was a common feature of asylums around the world.[3] It included the sounds of its staff, inmates, and objects. In Victorian asylums, 'the

---

[1] Report on the Lunatic Asylum at Colaba for the Year Ending 1852, GoB, GD, 1853/48, MSA, Mumbai.

[2] John Murray, *Handbook of the Bombay Presidency: With an Account of Bombay City, 1814–1883*, Second Edition (London: J Murray, 1881), p. 131.

[3] Dolly Mackinnon, 'Hearing Madness the Soundscape of the Asylum', in Catharine Coleborne and Dolly Mackinnon (eds.), *Madness in Australia: Histories, Heritage and the Asylum* (Queensland: University of Queensland Press, 2003), p. 79.

© The Author(s) 2018
S. A. Pinto, *Lunatic Asylums in Colonial Bombay*,
Mental Health in Historical Perspective,
https://doi.org/10.1007/978-3-319-94244-5_5

sensory environment ... was central to the management of the institution and the experience of the inmate', and this consideration informed the 'reform and modification of [its] architecture'.[4] Since the regulation of the aural environment was crucial to the management of asylums, this chapter seeks to reconstruct the soundscape of the colonial asylums in the Bombay Presidency. The factor that distinguished the asylum soundscapes in Bombay from other asylums in the world was the lack of 'regulation and regimentation' of the aural environment. The chapter particularly focuses on the padded room. The segregation of patients in separate boarded rooms started in the Bombay Presidency only in the mid-nineteenth century. Eventually, asylum staff converted these rooms into padded rooms. Superintendents in Bombay used it only for violent rather than noisy patients. Padded rooms eventually lost their significance for noise control, and superintendents even dismantled some of them.

The chapter examines the factors that contributed to ineffective sound management because the disorderly soundscape was further evidence of the failure of the asylum system as a colonial enterprise. The chapter argues that superintendents failed to achieve 'sonic hegemony'[5] within the asylum walls. For the colonial medical system to achieve aural hegemony, the regulation and regimentation of sound should have included a system of classification of patients based on propensity to create noise and proficiency in the English language.[6] The asylum superintendents, however, struggled to regulate 'noise', and Indian languages dominated the soundscape of the asylums all over the Presidency. Economic constraints and the nature of the asylum as a middle ground[7] restricted sonic hegemonization. The increasing 'regimentation and regulation' of the soundscape that characterized nineteenth-century asylums around the world[8] was not mirrored in Bombay's asylums. Surgeon James Cleghorn, Director General of

---

[4] Katherine Fennelly, 'Out of Sound, Out of Mind: Noise Control in Nineteenth-Century Lunatic Asylums in England and Ireland', *World Archaeology*, Vol. 46, 2014, No. 3, p. 417.

[5] Dolly Mackinnon argued that the domination of the English language, despite the language diversity among patients, was evidence of a continuing 'sonic imperialism'. The chapter uses the term 'sonic hegemony' to include both the process of hegemonizing the soundscape and the domination of the English language. The term 'sonic imperialism' when used here only refers to the domination of the English language. See Mackinnon, 'Hearing Madness', p. 78.

[6] Ibid.

[7] Richard White, *The Middle Ground: Indians, Empires, and Republics in the Great Lakes Region, 1650–1815* (Cambridge: Cambridge University Press, 1991).

[8] Mackinnon, 'Hearing Madness', p. 75.

the IMS noted that the 'the uproar and confusion' present in Indian asylums was in 'contrast to the quietness and order of a well-managed asylum'.[9] Finally, the chapter focuses on patients' voices that constituted the most manipulated feature of the chaotic asylum soundscape in the Bombay Presidency.

The aural environment in Bombay's asylums reflected a lack of classification based on sound and silence. Nineteenth-century Victorian asylums, in contrast, were a sight of order and classification, and the separation of 'noisy or disruptive' patients from recovering patients was of central importance to asylums in England.[10] Bombay's asylums did not have a system of segregation based on noise. In 1851, the Superintendent of the Colaba Lunatic Asylum elucidated that at the asylum all patients, 'male and female, the dark man and the white man, the noisy and the quiet' used the inner court and the garden.[11] Even 23 years later, superintendents failed to implement the classification of patients based on noise. On his visit to the Colaba Lunatic Asylum in 1874, Lord Napier of Magdala, Commander-in-Chief in India,[12] observed that though the asylum was 'very clean and well ventilated ... it was painful to see the violent insanes with those who were quiet and, perhaps, recovering'. The 'unhappy association' between the quiet and noisy patients, he commented, 'retarded, if not prevented' the cure of patients.[13] The lack of space in most asylums made classification extremely difficult and superintendents prioritized race, sex, class, and caste[14] as criteria for classification rather than the propensity of noise production.

Even asylum architecture did not facilitate the containing of sounds within the asylum. Architects in England and Ireland designed asylums to

---

[9] Note by the Director General, IMS, on the Reports of Lunatic Asylums under Local Governments and Administrations for the Year 1895, Medical Proceedings, Government of India, Home Department, Simla Records, September 1896, Nos. 65–90, NAI.

[10] Susan Piddock, *A Space of Their Own: The Archaeology of Nineteenth-Century Lunatic Asylums in Britain, South Australia and Tasmania* (New York: Springer, 2007), p. 39.

[11] From the Superintendent, Lunatic Asylum, Colaba, to the Secretary to the Medical Board, 21 June 1851, GoB, GD, 1851/15, MSA.

[12] https://www.britannica.com/biography/Robert-Napier-1st-Baron-Napier; accessed 5 October 2016.

[13] APR, 1873–1874, p. 21, NLS, Scotland.

[14] Waltraud Ernst, 'Madness and Colonial Spaces in British India', in L. Topp, James Moran and Jonathan Andrews (eds.), *Madness, Architecture and the Built Environment: Psychiatric Spaces in Historical Context* (New York, London: Routledge, 2007), p. 232.

ensure noise control.[15] Vaulted ceilings 'created a series of concave arches
... which concentrate[d] sound rather than scattering it'.[16] However, the
containment of sound was not a priority for superintendents in Bombay,
faced with other major defects and a stringent budget. Dr. Campbell,
Superintendent at the Colaba Lunatic Asylum, noted: 'A lesser evil [than
the other defects was] the absence of any medium in the flooring of the
upper storey to deaden the sound. There is nothing here but the bare
plank. The reverberation, in consequence, is excessive and in case of noise
it is heard not only all over the buildings but to a considerable distance
beyond them'.[17] Noise control was so hard to achieve that even passers-by
heard the sounds from the asylum.[18] The colonial asylum soundscape was
indeed a highly permeable one.

BOARDED AND PADDED ROOMS

The padded room, crucial to noise control in nineteenth-century asylums
elsewhere, failed to occupy a significant place in Bombay's asylums. In
other parts of the world, asylum staff isolated patients in darkened or quiet
rooms to maintain effective sound control.[19] Padded rooms became
increasingly popular in the second half of the nineteenth century as a
replacement for mechanical restraint.[20] The Colaba Lunatic Asylum had
the first boarded room built in 1847.[21] The room had a common roof and
was divided into six cells; it was 'built on arches and [had] no windows, air
being admitted by minute perforations in the floor, and small apertures in
the upper part of their front and back walls'. The black cells measured 'ten
feet long, nine and a half feet broad and twelve and half feet in height'.[22]
The cells were located on the south eastern corner of the grounds. The
Visitors to the Colaba Lunatic Asylum noted that superintendents only

[15] Fennelly, 'Out of Sound, Out of Mind', p. 424.
[16] Ibid., p. 425.
[17] Report on the Lunatic Asylum at Colaba for the Year Ending 1852, GoB, GD, 1853/48,
MSA.
[18] John Murray, *Handbook of the Bombay Presidency*, p. 131.
[19] Fennelly, 'Out of Sound, Out of Mind', p. 422.
[20] John Conolly, *The Treatment of the Insane Without Mechanical Restraints* (London:
Smith, Elder and Co., 1856), p. 42.
[21] Official records use the term 'padded room' from the late 1860s onwards.
[22] Report on the Lunatic Asylum at Colaba for the Year Ending 1852, GoB, GD, 1853/48,
MSA.

occasionally used these rooms.[23] When Dr. Campbell superintended the Colaba Lunatic Asylum, he built two additional boarded rooms for European patients. These boarded rooms were located between the dispensary and infirmary.[24] In the second half of the century, asylum records only refer to padded rooms; therefore it is likely that asylum agencies eventually converted these boarded rooms to padded rooms.[25] The Ratnagiri Lunatic Asylum plan reveals the building of padded rooms for each ward: male, female, and the criminal ward.[26] By 1903, the government of Bombay, however, acknowledged that only the asylums at Colaba and Naupada had padded rooms.[27] The padded rooms at Ratnagiri and Dharwar either fell into disuse or asylum staff used them for other purposes.[28]

Superintendents used the padded room for violent patients rather than noisy ones. They used the 'dark boarded cell' for treating 'violent and unruly patients' who were kept there 'until the excitement subside[d]'.[29] Superintendents and Visitors sent patients from *mofussil* asylums to the Colaba Lunatic Asylum if they needed incarceration in a padded cell. In 1871, the Visitors petitioned for the transfer of an extremely 'dangerous and violent' criminal patient, Geelam Hussain, from the Poona Lunatic Asylum. The Visitors requested for Geelam's transfer to the Colaba Lunatic Asylum that had a padded room.[30] Asylum staff used 'violence' rather than 'noise' as the criterion for incarceration in a padded room. They believed that such rooms served to manage patients with 'destructive habits' or patients who were 'refractory', 'uproarious', or 'dangerous'.[31] Superintendents in India acknowledged that the poor regulation of noise was peculiar to Indian asylums.

[23] Extract from the Remarks recorded by the Visitors, 12 September 1859, GoB, GD, 1859/24, MSA.

[24] Report on the Lunatic Asylum at Colaba for the Year Ending 1852, GoB, GD, 1853/48, MSA.

[25] Extract from the Proceeding of the Visitors of the Lunatic Asylum, Poona, 4 September 1871, GoB, GD, 1871/34, MSA.

[26] See Fig. 5.1.

[27] From A.M.T. Jackson, Acting Secretary to Government of Bombay, to the Secretary to the Government of India, 27 June 1903, Home Department, Medical Proceedings, Simla Records, GoB, GD, 1903/57, MSA.

[28] APR, 1874–1875, p. 18, NLS.

[29] APR, 1873–1874, p. 4, NLS.

[30] Extract from the Proceeding of the Visitors of the Lunatic Asylum, Poona, 4 September 1871, GoB, GD, 1871/34, MSA.

[31] From John Scott, Secretary to the Medical Board, to the Bombay Medical Board Office, 3 June 1851, GoB, GD 1852/10, MSA; APR, 1873–1874, pp. 20–21, 23, NLS.

Dr. A.W. Overbeck-Wright, Superintendent of the lunatic asylum at Agra, discussed the lack of control over noise in the colonial asylum soundscape. In his book *Mental Derangements in India*, he elaborated on the lack of regulation on the sensory environment in Indian lunatic asylums by comparing the use of the padded room in English and Indian asylums. In Britain, he explained, staff considered a noisy patient 'to upset the whole place'. In order to control such patients they were 'shut up in the padded room, where he can shout certainly, but no one hears the music but himself'.[32] In contrast, he observed that in Indian asylums, 'if a patient shouts he is left alone, or at most a sedative is given if he requires it, and [the patients is] allowed to shout to his heart's content without the other patients in any way being affected'.[33] In the twentieth century, superintendents felt that padded rooms were not required in India, since a tiny dose of 'suphanol or other sedatives was sufficient to tame and quiet the most unruly'.[34] Superintendents used the padded cell only occasionally and under the 'strictest supervision'.[35]

The materials used in Bombay's padded cells were indicative of its use as a means of restraint for violent patients rather than noisy patients. Initially, the 'boarded room' was made of a 'succession of tubes made of tiles … laid in parallel rows, with layers of mortar'.[36] Tarred canvas provided extra padding for the room; eventually, however, doctors objected to its use. Engineers replaced tarred canvas with oil painted canvas. Towards the end of the nineteenth century, government engineers devised cost-effective padded cells for Indian asylums.[37] These cells were made of 'good choir' mattresses nailed to the seven-foot wall and

[32] A.W. Overbeck-Wright, *Mental Derangements in India: Its Symptoms and Treatment* (Calcutta and Simla: Thacker, Spink and Co., 1912), p. 326.

[33] Ibid.

[34] Ibid; W.G.H. Henderson Superintendent, Poona Lunatic Asylum, to the Personal Asst. with the Surgeon General, Government of Bombay, 18 July 1904, GoB, GD, 1907/81, MSA.

[35] W.G.H. Henderson, Superintendent, Poona Lunatic Asylum to the Personal Asst. with the Surgeon General, Government of Bombay, 18 July 1904, GoB, GD, 1907/81, MSA.

[36] Report on the Lunatic Asylum at Colaba for the Year Ending 1852, GoB, GD, 1853/48, MSA.

[37] From the Executive Engineer to the Superintending Engineer, 6 June 1903, GoB, GD, 1903/57, MSA.

to the floor. A sailcloth painted with oil paint up to three feet covered the mattresses, since government engineers 'found [that height] sufficient to prevent fouling of the upper unpainted canvas by the lunatics'.[38] At the Narotamdas Madhavdas Lunatic Asylum, Thana, engineers used leather instead of plain sailcloth because it was more durable.[39] In 1904, Miss Shepherd, the Chaplain of the Colaba Lunatic Asylum, who worked for Church of England, described how she could hear patients through the padded rooms, which she referred to as the 'wild beast den'. She asked the *ayah* to open the shutters to let in a little light for the 'poor Jewess' who was 'shouting and crying with terror'.[40] The padded rooms in Bombay's asylums were poorly sound-proofed unlike padded rooms in Britain. Along with the poor quality of soundproofing, Bombay's superintendents had other problems with padded rooms (Fig. 5.1).

The cost of maintaining padded rooms and their poor durability made them unpopular with superintendents. As one superintendent explained, padded rooms in Indian asylums were 'objectionable' because they 'easily gave cover to vermin'.[41] The padded room at the Ahmedabad Lunatic Asylum was dismantled 'owing to its moth-eaten condition and to its never having been required'.[42] The Superintendent at Poona reasoned that the padded rooms at the Poona Lunatic Asylum were 'useless' and he had them converted into 'ordinary cells'.[43] Even several years after the establishment of the Central Lunatic Asylum at Yerawada, there was no provision for padded rooms.[44] The cost-ineffectiveness and high maintenance of padded rooms caused their exclusion and scant use as an architectural feature of Bombay's asylums.

[38] From the Executive Engineer to the Superintending Engineer, 6 June 1903, GoB, GD, 1903/57, MSA.

[39] From the Acting Superintending Engineer to the Secretary to the Government, 10 June 1903, PWD, GoB, GD, 1903/58, MSA.

[40] From Miss Mary Shepherd to the Governor in Council, 31 May 1904, GoB, GD, 1904/57, MSA.

[41] APR, 1874–1875, p. 18, NLS.

[42] APR, 1915, p. 1, NLS.

[43] APR, 1895, p. 1, NLS.

[44] From the Surgeon General with the Government of Bombay to the Secretary to the Government, 25 June 1918, Poona, Triennial Report of the Lunatic Asylum under the Government of Bombay for the Year 1915–1917, p. 1, NLS.

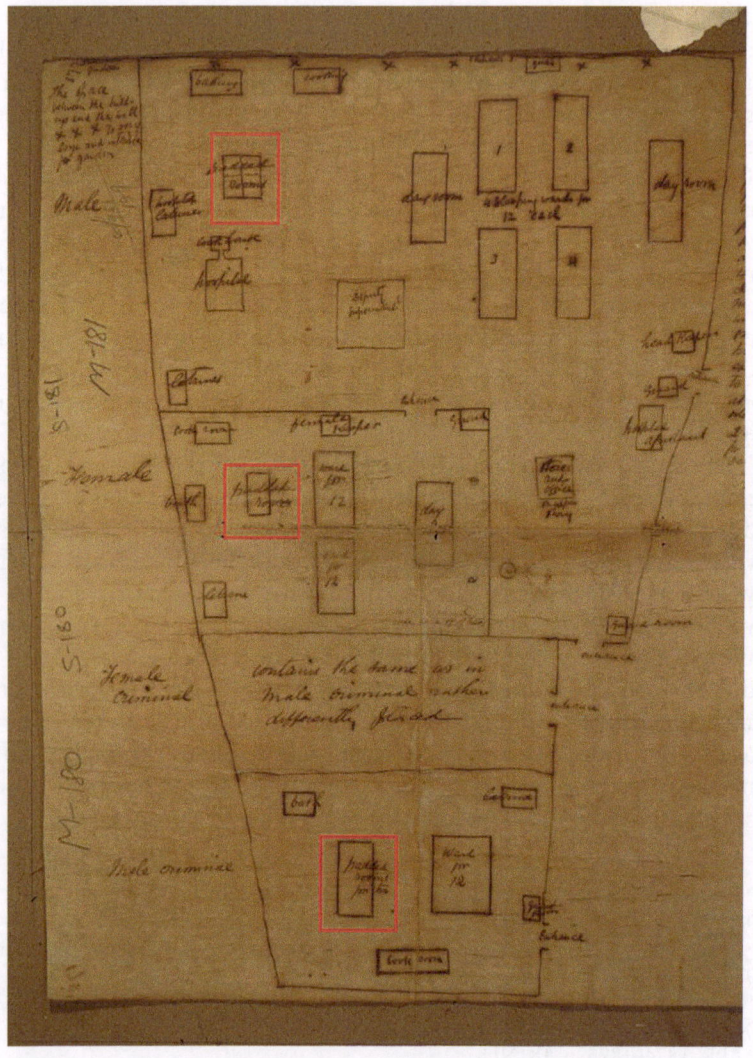

Fig. 5.1 Padded rooms at Ratnagiri Lunatic Asylum. (Source: Plan of the Ratnagiri Lunatic Asylum, GoB, GD, 1886/58, MSA)

SOUND MANAGEMENT

The segregation of patients based on 'sound and noise' was a rare phenomenon in Bombay's asylums. Interestingly, this was a time when in Victorian asylums a 'refined system of classification was becoming the heart of a model asylum's operational arrangements'.[45] Colonial asylums, by contrast, fell short of achieving this ideal. Even at the main asylum of the Presidency at Colaba, asylum staff classified only female patients based on sound and noise. Dr. Campbell described the classification in this way: 'The Europeans and females each are divided into two classes, of these the quiet, cleanly and convalescent occupy the upper wards ... and the noisy dirty and destructive the lower'.[46] By 1870, Visitors commented that the whole system of classification at Colaba Lunatic Asylum was 'defective ... [since] the dirty and foulmouthed ... [were] often associated with the harmless and inoffensive insane'.[47] Several factors contributed to the deficient arrangements for noise control and classification.

The colonial asylum was particularly noisy at night, when even patients complained of the noise. The European patients at Colaba blamed the Indian patients for the noisy environment within the asylum. Private Lennon, a patient in the European ward, reported to the Coroner who was investigating the case of a patient who committed suicide: 'The horrors of the night in the Colaba Lunatic Asylum were enough to drive a sane person mad, and it was difficult to get sleep from the horrid shoutings of the natives and the banging of doors'.[48] The Indian patients, however, blamed the subordinate staff for the noises within the asylum. The sounds of the conversations of staff during the night disturbed patients. Sajan Curim, a patient at the Colaba Lunatic Asylum, in a letter to the government complained about the noise created by subordinate staff. He objected that the noise at night was 'intolerable, recurring every two hours, especially of the peons and the *Halalcores* (sweepers) who talk loudly'.[49] In the *mofussil* asylums, the shortage of staff only added to the

[45] Ernst, 'Madness and Colonial Spaces', p. 55.

[46] Report on the Lunatic Asylum at Colaba for the Year Ending 1852, GoB, GD, 1853/48, MSA.

[47] From the Visitors of the Colaba Lunatic Asylum to the Secretary to the Government of Bombay, JD, 23 August 1870, GoB, GD, 1871/34, MSA

[48] From the Coroner of Bombay to the Secretary to the Government, JD, 15 March 1871, GoB, GD, 1871/34, MSA.

[49] From Sajan Curim to the Secretary to the Government of Bombay, 16 October 1893, GoB, GD, 1893/75, MSA.

poor regulation of loud noises, especially at night. At the Dharwar Lunatic Asylum, there was no supervision at night; the asylum had about 20 patients managed by two warders. The attendants would lock up the asylum at night and leave.[50] By 1876, the superintendent moved the quieter patients to dayrooms at night with their keepers. While superintendents complained of the lack of quiet spaces within the asylum, they often used sound to facilitate supervision.

Asylum staff employed 'silence and sound' to maintain surveillance and discipline.[51] Superintendents in Bombay used mechanical restraints because of the sounds this created, despite its increasing unpopularity over the nineteenth century. Dr. Niven, Superintendent at the Colaba Lunatic Asylum, put iron chains on one patient's legs even though he was a 'quiet' patient. The noise of the iron chains, explained Dr. Niven, would 'direct the constant attention of the warders' to him.[52] Dr. Niven used iron chains to monitor that patient, since he was a criminal patient who had attempted to escape from prison and the asylum. The Medical Board, however, on hearing of this incident, reprimanded him for resorting to the use of mechanical restraint on the 'quiet' patient; the following year the superintendent removed the chains.[53] Among the sounds that facilitated supervision, the sound of the *ghury* (clock) resounded at regular intervals. The sound of the clock helped warders who could not read time. Warder Megha Purajee, who acted as a witness in a patient suicide case, explained that he 'knew it was 3 Am because [he] had just heard the ghury strike'.[54] Similar to asylums in Australia, 'the bell' played an important role in regulating asylum life. At the Ratnagiri Lunatic Asylum, a bell served to indicate to staff and patients the hours for meals.[55] Asylum staff used the stimulation of sound for regulating asylum practices. Sound and noise were characteristic of the colonial asylum soundscape, leaving little space for silence (Fig. 5.2).

Amusements also included the creation and accommodation of sounds. In the 1870s, superintendents introduced music to Bombay's asylum

[50] From the Superintendent, Dharwar Lunatic Asylum to the Secretary of Government, 2 December 1870, JD, GoB, GD, 1870/9, MSA.

[51] Mackinnon, 'Hearing Madness', p. 76.

[52] APR, 1873–1874, p. 4, NLS.

[53] APR, 1873–1874, p. 21, NLS.

[54] Information taken on oath from Megha Purajee, 6 March 1871, GoB, GD, 1871/34, MSA.

[55] See Fig. 5.2.

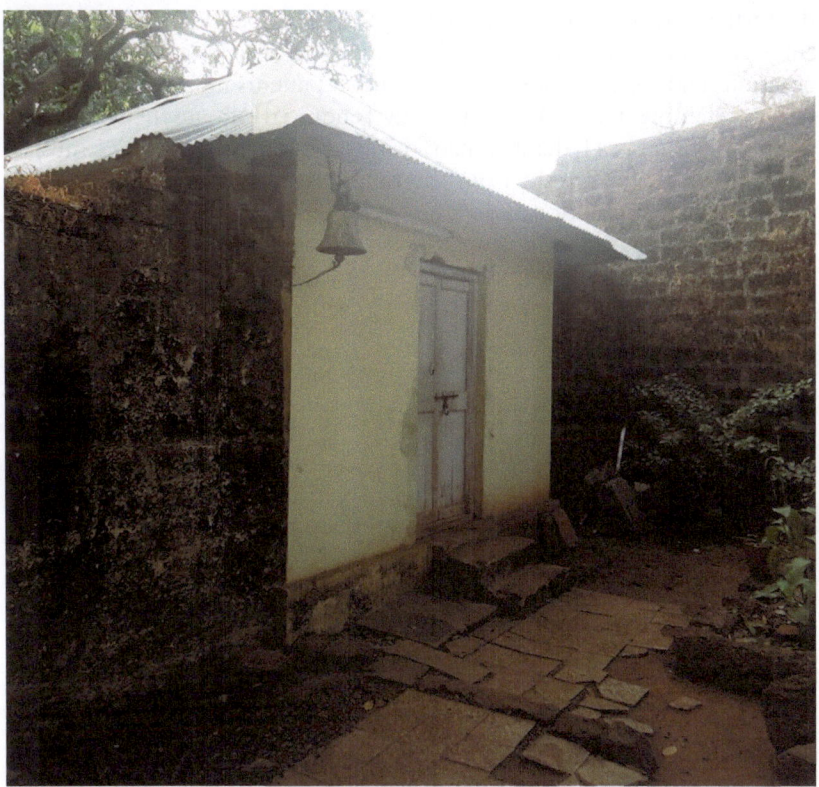

Fig. 5.2 The bell at the Ratnagiri Asylum (Ratnagiri Mental Hospital). The bell is attached to a small intermediary room where staff bring food to the patients. Patients then carry the food over to the dining area. (Source: Author's Photograph, November 2014)

soundscape. Dolly Mackinnon argued that in Australian asylums superintendents used music as medicine and a means of 'influencing the unsound mind'.[56] Likewise, Bombay's superintendents considered music to be 'conducive to the health and comfort' of the patients.[57] Music filled

---

[56] Dolly Mackinnon, '"Jolly and Fond of Singing": The Gendered Nature of Musical Entertainment in Queensland Mental Institutions, c1870-1937', in Coleborne and Mackinnon, *Madness in Australia: Histories, Heritage and the Asylum*, p. 160.

[57] APR, 1898, p. 9, NLS.

the asylum environment as 'native musicians were periodically engaged to entertain and amuse patients'. Musicians were usually called on special occasions and superintendents reported that patients not only appreciated the entertainment but also 'constantly [enquired] about their return'.[58] The new asylum at Hyderabad had 'drums and banjos' and native musical instruments available right from the time it was established in 1871. Sir Cowasji Jehangir also donated a musical box to the asylum in 1876.[59] The Ahmedabad Lunatic Asylum was the only other asylum that had musical instruments for patients' amusement.[60] Musical instruments were issued in the evenings, 'two or three times a week: some [patients] play[ed], while other dance[d] and caper[ed] around … [it made] them happy and cheerful'.[61] Pets also added to the asylum soundscape, as superintendents kept pigs, cats, dogs, fowl, monkeys, and deer for the amusement of patients.[62] Lunatic asylums in Bombay were noisy sites as superintendents failed to regulate and regiment the soundscape.

Superintendents also could never secure the dominance of the English language within the asylum soundscape or 'sonic imperialism'[63] within Bombay's asylums. Local languages continued to dominate the asylum soundscape. In comparison, in Australian and Irish asylums, despite the diversity in asylum patient population, sonic imperialism was in operation with 'English forming the dominant spoken language'.[64] However, in India, even superintendents had to learn the local language or appoint assistants for translation. When the discussion of a new asylum site for Sindh began in 1862, Superintendent Niven objected to the asylum being built at Larkhana because it was too isolated for superintendents who would have to stay long enough to 'acquire the language' and 'be acquainted with the patients'.[65] When Bombay's superintendents objected to the government proposal of bringing in an expert from England to manage the asylums of the Presidency, the inability of

[58] APR, 1898, p. 9, NLS.
[59] APR, 1877, p. 23, NLS.
[60] APR, 1882, p. 6, NLS.
[61] APR, 1874–1875, p. 29, NLS.
[62] Report on the Lunatic Asylum at Colaba for the Year Ending 1852, GoB, GD, 1853/48, MSA; APR, 1877, p. 23, NLS.
[63] Mackinnon, 'Hearing Madness', p. 80.
[64] Fennelly, 'Out of Sound, Out of Mind', p. 427.
[65] From the Superintendent, Lunatic Asylum, Larkhana, to Captain J. Leith, 15 July 1862, GoB, GD, 1862–1864/15, MSA.

superintendents to understand the language of Indian patients was stated as a significant reason why a 'novice from England'[66] would useless in an Indian asylum. Superintendent B.B. Grayfoot noted: 'It would take him [the expert] six years to learn all the different languages in his big asylum'. Furthermore, he explained that Indian patients preferred 'attendants who speak his [their] language and understand his [their] ways'.[67] In Poona, the Surgeon General recommended that a Hospital Assistant serve 'as a means of communication with the native patients'.[68] The local Indian subordinate staff had only a sparse understanding of English.[69]

Asylum staff used local Indian languages even for official communication within the asylum. The use of local languages in Bombay's asylum contrasted with the Australian and Irish asylums where English was the official language. In Australian and Irish asylums, rules were composed in English for patients and staff. Katherine Fennelly has argued that the domination of English was a form of 'cultural colonialism'.[70] In Bombay's asylums, however, local languages dominated official communication. Superintendents were willing to negotiate the use of Indian languages, since it would persuade Indians to use the asylum. The medical class made a recommendation to the government in the 1860's to establish district asylums, since they believed that Indians would be more willing to use the asylum if staff spoke their language.[71] Superintendents also negotiated the use of Indian language with their staff. In 1875, Superintendent P. Murphy wrote to the government seeking permission for the translation of the General Rules of the Asylum into Marathi[72] for 'guidance of the overseers,

[66] Letter from Lt. Col. J.W.T Anderson, Superintendent, Lunatic Asylum, Ahmedabad, to the Personal Asst. to the Surgeon General with the Government of Bombay, 10 July 1904, GoB, GD 1907/81, MSA.

[67] Letter from B.B. Grayfoot, Superintendent, Lunatic Asylum, Dharwar, to the Personal Asst. to the Asst. to the Surgeon General with the Government of Bombay, 10 August 1904, GoB, GD, 1907/81, MSA.

[68] Letter from Surgeon General G. Bainbridge, Surgeon General with the Government of Bombay, 10 July 1899, GoB, GD, 1900/62, MSA.

[69] From Miss Mary Shepherd, W.C.C. Fort, 21 May 1904, GoB, GD, 1904/57, MSA.

[70] Fennelly, 'Out of Sound, Out of Mind', p. 426.

[71] Medical Department Circular, GD Vol.15, No. 555, 1862–1864, MSA, in Shruti Kapila, 'The Making of Colonial Psychiatry, Bombay Presidency, 1849–1940', PhD Thesis, School of Oriental and African Studies, University of London, 2002, p. 61.

[72] Marathi was the local language of the area that comprises modern-day Maharashtra State in India.

warders and all others employed in the asylum',[73] after which the government also translated the General Rules into Gujarati[74] for the use of the Superintendent at Ahmedabad.[75] The Government Central Press printed these translations.[76] Superintendents negotiated the use of Indian languages with staff to meet a 'specific end':[77] better management of the asylum. The domination of Indian languages within the asylum soundscape is indicative of the nature of the asylum as a middle ground.

The lack of control over the aural environment in Bombay's asylums was the result of colonial perceptions of Indians. Public asylums in England reflected the 'quiet tenor' of 'middle-class domesticity' that characterized Victorian streets.[78] By contrast, colonial medical staff in India thought that Indian patients adjusted well to noise. In Bombay's asylums, restrictions on sounds were therefore relaxed. Colonial superintendents perceived Indian society to be 'noisy' and so they maintained the asylum soundscape according to that perception. The lunatic asylum at Colaba stood 'in close proximity to a crowded village with all its disagreeable concomitants of noise and dirt and to the lighthouse with its exciting accompaniments of night lamps and signal guns'. Dr. Campbell complained that the sounds from the village and lighthouse had a 'disturbing influence' and was 'productive of serious injury' on the inmates. The noise, he believed, had a more serious impact on his European patients compared to Indian patients. The 'natives', he explained, 'appear[ed] ... to become soon reconciled to it'.[79] The superintendents' notion that noise had little impact on Indian patients meant that classification of patients based on 'noise' never became a priority.

Classification between the 'quiet and the violent'[80] was considered ideal and beneficial but was difficult to maintain due to overcrowding and the

---

[73] From the Superintendent, Colaba Lunatic Asylum, to the Deputy Surgeon General of Bombay, 29 December 1874, GoB, GD, 1875/38, MSA.

[74] Gujarati was the local language of the area that comprises modern-day Gujarat state in India.

[75] From the Surgeon General, IMD, to the Secretary to the Government, 30 April 1875, GoB, GD, 1875/38, MSA.

[76] Government Resolution, 17 September 1875, Bombay Castle, GoB, GD, 1875/38, MSA.

[77] White, *The Middle Ground*, p. 51.

[78] Fennelly, 'Out of Sound, Out of Mind', p. 417.

[79] Report on the Lunatic Asylum at Colaba for the Year Ending 1852, GoB, GD, 1853/48, MSA.

[80] From John Scott, Secretary to the Medical Board, to the Bombay Medical Board Office, 3 June 1851, GoB, GD 1852/10, MSA.

spatial configuration of asylum buildings. On 6 December 1899, Surgeon General G. Bainbridge visited the Colaba Lunatic Asylum; he described the arrangement of patients there. The asylum, he said, 'was clean and efficiently supervised'; however, 'the arrangement of the buildings [did] not permit of the proper grouping of the different forms of insanity, or the complete separation of noisy and violent patients'.[81] The Ratnagiri Lunatic Asylum had no proper accommodation for 'excited and noisy patients' and the existing cross cell arrangement did not ensure 'proper supervision'.[82] The Superintendent at Dharwar complained about a similar condition at his asylum, concerning patient classification in 1874:

> The mild and gentle monomaniac recovering to sanity is compelled to asso-
> ciate with the foul and obscene howling maniac who constantly shocks every
> sense of decency.[83]

Even two years later, the asylum staff made no improvements in the system of classification of noisy and quiet patients at Dharwar. Superintendent C. J. Sylvester in 1877 reported the lack of arrangements and an urgent need for 'classification and separation of patients who are partially recovered from others who are filthy in their habits, noisy and obscene'.[84] By 1899, the condition at the Dharwar Lunatic Asylum had worsened, and even juveniles were associating with noisy and violent adults.[85] The classification of noisy patients remained a challenge for colonial superintendents.

Economic constraints limited the efforts of superintendents in 'regimenting and regulating'[86] the asylum soundscape. Dr. Henderson, Superintendent of the Poona Lunatic Asylum, complained that the most important task of separating 'the insane who… [were] quietening down' was obstructed by 'the usual financial difficulty [that] steps in and debars officers making recommendations which they know would be futile'.[87] Furthermore, medicines that aided the sedating of noisy patients were often too expensive for the asylum budget. Superintendent J.P. Barry

---

[81] APR, 1899, p. 14, NLS.
[82] APR, 1899, p. 1, NLS.
[83] APR, 1874–1875, p. 18, NLS.
[84] APR, 1876, p. 18, NLS.
[85] APR, 1899, p. 14, NLS.
[86] Mackinnon, 'Hearing Madness', p. 75.
[87] W.G.H. Henderson, Superintendent, Poona Lunatic Asylum, to the Personal Asst. with the Surgeon General, Government of Bombay, 18 July 1904, GoB, GD, 1907/81, MSA.

stated that at the Narotamdas Madhavdas Lunatic Asylum, 'One of the commonest drugs used to quieten the violent and sleepless ... was struck out of the list as if it meant a treasonable attack on the budget'.[88] Limited by a strict budget, superintendents either left patients to 'shout to their heart's content'[89] or applied other methods to control their noisy behaviour.

The superintendents devised practical ways to manage noisy patients. They used employment as one of the principal methods to exert control over patient noises. Surgeon Holmstead, Superintendent of the Hyderabad Lunatic Asylum, explained: 'There is no counter-irritant equal to bodily labour'.[90] Superintendents advocated patient labour since it produced a tranquillizing effect on the patient's body and mind. Superintendent Niven of the Colaba Lunatic Asylum, in the Annual Asylum Report for 1873–1874, explained:

> It has several times been brought to my notice how well all the noisy patients sleep when they are employed for three or four hours in the afternoon, carrying sand or mud for garden or reclamation purposes for the foreshore when there is ebb tide. My firm conviction is that if the asylum had 20–30 acres of cultivable land attached to it the cures would be doubled.[91]

Superintendents laboured patients to exhaustion in order to manage the asylum soundscape. While patient labour reduced the volume of sound within the asylum to some extent, superintendents also employed patients to manage sounds coming from outside the asylum. The asylum at Hyderabad was situated close to the public road and the 'noise occasioned by carriages and other conveyances, and ... people passing ... was easily heard in the female ward making them frightened and troublesome'. Therefore, using patient labour, the superintendent built a wall 11 feet high around the entire quarter. The wall provided some privacy and quietened the female ward to some extent. The results were greatly beneficial to the female patients and it was 'manifest in [their] subdued demeanour and improved behaviour', while earlier, it was 'impossible to keep them

---

[88] From Superintendent J.P Barry to the Personal Asst. to the Surgeon General with the Government of Bombay, 25 June 1904, GoB, GD, 1907/81, MSA.

[89] Overbeck-Wright, *Mental Derangements in India*, p. 326.

[90] APR, 1874–1875, p. 26, NLS.

[91] APR, 1873–1874, p. 4, NLS.

quiet'.[92] Superintendents thus justified the labouring of patients based on the notion that it helped control noisy patients.

Superintendents adhered to a gendered division of labour when regulating the noise of patients. Superintendents usually employed men in construction work, manual labour, or agriculture.[93] They believed grain grinding to be particularly useful for treating noisy women. At the Sir Cowasji Jehangir Lunatic Asylum at Hyderabad, the Superintendent reported, in 1873, that women were more difficult to manage compared to the men. Once the superintendent introduced women to grain grinding, he observed a change in them. They became 'orderly and quiet' and were 'blithely singing at their tasks'. He reported that there was such an improvement in them that sometimes it was difficult to tell that they were 'really demented'.[94] Superintendents considered labour and noise management intrinsically connected.

Despite such efforts of superintendents to manage noise through labour, Bombay's asylums gained a reputation for their unruly soundscapes. By the latter decades of the nineteenth century when the government began discussing plans for a new site for an asylum in Poona, one site was considered unsuitable on grounds that 'noise in the asylum might disturb the employees of finance offices' and other offices in the vicinity.[95] On the one hand, superintendents wanted the asylums to be centrally located and easily accessible by the railways. On the other, the poor regulation of sound and noise from the asylum presented an obstacle to this preference. From the early twentieth century, the government built asylums in more isolated locations to avoid causing disturbances to the surrounding localities. The Narotamdas Madhavdas Lunatic Asylum at Naupada, built in 1902, was so isolated that the superintendent complained about its location.[96] The inability to regulate noise within the asylum influenced the choice for new asylum sites in the twentieth century.

---

[92] APR, 1873–1874, p. 46, NLS.
[93] APR, 1873–1874, p. 4; APR, 1873–1874, p. 46, NLS.
[94] APR, 1873–1874, p. 30, NLS.
[95] Report of the Committee Assembled under the Government Resolution, General Department, No. 951, 'To Select a Suitable Site for the New Lunatic Asylum at Poona', 17 April 1869, GoB, GD, 1870/9, MSA.
[96] Letter from Lt. Col. Barry, Superintendent Colaba Lunatic Asylum to the Personal Asst. to the Surgeon General with the Government of Bombay, 25 June 1904, GoB, GD, 1907/81, MSA.

PATIENTS' VOICES

'the most unfortunate legacy of the Age of the Asylum was the silencing of the patient'. Petteri Pietikainen[97]

Patients' voices were an important part of the asylum soundscape. This section examines the management of patients' voices and their significance to the asylum soundscape. Within asylum walls, the staff evaluated, interpreted, and manipulated patients' voices for their diagnostic and evidential value. The manipulation and interpretation of patients' voices were essential to managing the soundscape, because the 'mad both articulated their condition and were defined as such by others, through interpretive hearing'.[98] Patients' voices were thus extremely important in identifying their insanity. Most patients in Indian asylums came from the poorest section of the society. It was difficult for superintendents to gain information about patients since they found patients' relatives difficult to trace or they were 'ignorant and uneducated'.[99] This lack of information meant that doctors had to depend on the descriptive roll on the medical certificate. Police constables filled in these descriptive rolls on the lunacy certificates based on 'the statement of the lunatic while still insane', and interestingly, these descriptions provided 'not only the history and habits but also the cause of his insanity'.[100] A patient's speech, then, was decisive evidence of his own insanity.

On committal to the asylum, a patient's speech and silence were evaluated, interpreted, and manipulated to serve the diagnostic process. Dr. Overbeck-Wright highlighted the importance of the patient's speech in the diagnostic process:

> Speech ... is closely connected with all the mental processes that it is unusually implicated in the course of insanity ... . The mental condition is often indicated by the character of speech.[101]

Dr. Overbeck-Wright recommended that superintendents closely observe both speech and 'silence' as a means of evaluating them.[102] The wards of

---

[97] Petteri Pietikainen, *Madness: A History* (London and New York: Routledge Taylor and Francis Group, 2015), p. 145.

[98] Mackinnon, 'Hearing Madness', p. 76.

[99] Report of the Indian Hemp Drugs Commission, 1894–1895, Vol. 2, p. 232, NLS.

[100] Report of the Indian Hemp Drugs Commission, 1894–1895, Vol. 2, p. 232, NLS.

[101] A.W. Overbeck-Wright, *Lunacy in India* (London: Bailliere, Tindall and Cox, 1921), p. 53.

[102] Ibid., p. 188.

the eastern wing at the Colaba Lunatic Asylum with patients needing the most attention came under the 'immediate eye and ear of the superintendent'. Furthermore, the windows of the ward opened towards the superintendent's bungalow so that 'he could hear the voices of patients even when they conversed in a moderate tone'.[103] Dr. Campbell reported the symptoms of insanity related to speech that he observed in his patients:

> Some manifested curious perversities of feeling and sensation, one never spoke, another was never silent … to detail all the strange manifestations of diseased intellectual and moral constitution, which have been observed during the year.[104]

After the superintendents heard patients' voices, they then interpreted them. While evaluating and interpreting the patient's voice, they closely monitored the character of the patient's speech and silence. Dr. Overbeck-Wright cautioned superintendents about relying too much on patients' statements and recommended that they make conclusions based on their own 'observations, reasoning and medical examination … to distinguish what is true and false'.[105]

The case notes of Dr. Maxwell, who superintended the Colaba Lunatic Asylum in 1814, also provide evidence for the centrality of the diagnostic value of speech:

> [Name]: Gopal Parab
> 15th September: He was outrageous for twelve months after his admission. Since then he has been **tolerably sober and quiet**. He is at present pretty **coherent in his talk**. And in answers to questions put, says that he belongs to Bancoat and has relations there. Seems perfectly **quiet and harmless.**
> 25th October: Appetite good, **has been quiet**, since last report.
> 18th April: Has been **perfectly sober and quiet** since my getting charge of the hospital, and is now in good health.[106]

---

[103] Report on the Lunatic Asylum at Colaba for the Year Ending 1852, GoB, GD, 1853/48, MSA.
[104] Report on the Lunatic Asylum at Colaba for the Year Ending 1852, GoB, GD, 1853/48, MSA.
[105] Overbeck-Wright, *Lunacy in India*, p. 188.
[106] From Asst. Surgeon J.A. Maxwell to the Chief Secretary to the Government of Bombay, 4 June 1814, GoB, PDD, 1814/368, MSA. Text highlighted for emphasis.

Speech and silence thus became a yardstick to evaluate the mental condition of patients. Gopal's 'quietness' was interpreted as an index of improvement of his mental health. Paradoxically, in another patient, Shaikh Curim, his 'quietness' was interpreted as a specific type of insanity. The Superintendent diagnosed him as an 'idiot':

> [Name]: Shaik Curim
> 15th September 1813: Unable to walk, sullen, **seldom noisy and as seldom answer[s]** when spoken to
> 25th October 1813: Has been **quiet** during the month
> 25th November 1813: **Speaks oftener; yet still slow in answering** when spoken to.
> 25th January 1814: Not once violent or noisy in the last month
> 25th February 1814: **Still quiet** and harmless
> 18th April 1814: From **the stupid, dull and quiet state** that he always is in ... I am inclined to believe that **he is more of an idiot** than a maniac.[107]

Superintendents carefully evaluated patients' speech and silence, as they perceived it as indications of certain types of insanity.

Superintendents commonly used a list of set phrases to evaluate a patient's silence or speech. They used these phrases in the diagnostic process to define symptoms of a patient's insanity. 'Incoherence of speech' or talking 'nonsense' were common signs of insanity.[108] Conversely, they considered 'coherence of speech' and the ability to 'answer rationally' as signs of improvement. If a patient refused to answer the superintendent or reply to his questions or even if he answered slowly, the superintendent attributed that to his mental condition.[109] In one case, the superintendent reported improvement when the friends of a Muslim patient, Haji Ali, brought to his notice that 'he [Haji Ali] could repeat his prayers in a more distinct manner than when last seen by them'.[110] Superintendents made patients speak in order to gather information and evidence of their own insanity.

[107] From Asst. Surgeon J.A. Maxwell to the Chief Secretary to the Government of Bombay, 4 June 1814, GoB, PDD, 1814/368, MSA. Text highlighted for emphasis.
[108] Report of the Indian Hemp Drugs Commission, 1894–1895, Vol. 2, p. 193, NLS.
[109] From Asst. Surgeon J.A. Maxwell to the Chief Secretary to the Government, 4 June 1814, GoB, PDD, 1814/368, MSA.
[110] From Asst. Surgeon J.A. Maxwell to the Chief Secretary to the Government of Bombay, 4 June 1814, GoB, PDD, 1814/368, MSA.

Doctors also assessed patients based on the 'audiation they heard in their heads'.[111] They considered aural hallucinations the most common form of hallucination. Such hallucinations, they believed, were most 'pronounced at night'.[112] Patients suffering from these hallucinations were 'heard carrying on conversations with, or pouring forth volleys of abuse on, some invisible being'.[113] Doctors frequently reported patients muttering or talking to themselves. Dr. Maxwell's case notes record two patients, Shaik Ahmed and 'a robust Musalman', who were often found muttering to themselves.[114] A Sedee[115] patient at the Cowasji Jehangir Lunatic Asylum, Hyderabad, who was unwilling to work, would often ask asylum staff if they thought he was a *cooly*. The Superintendent recorded that the Sedee 'would talk for hours aloud to imaginary people'.[116] Doctors even examined aural hallucinations to ascertain various 'social causes' of insanity.[117] The Superintendent at Hyderabad explained that 'religious enthusiasm, unsuccessful litigation, commercial vicissitudes and unhappy domestic relations' were reflected in the prevailing hallucinations. While patients' voices were significant to the diagnostic process, they also served other purposes in the asylum.

Patients' voices had evidential value. Government agencies and asylum staff often asked patients to act as witnesses when there was an escape, suicide, murder, or negligence. In 1853, Dudley, a European patient at the Colaba Lunatic Asylum, escaped. Asylum staff questioned the patients about Dudley. One patient reported seeing him 'take a suit of white clothes out of his box the day before his escape'.[118] When enquiries were conducted, the voices of the warders and European patients had more value than those of the Indian patients. During 1870–1871, there were

[111] Mackinnon, 'Hearing Madness', p. 77.
[112] Overbeck -Wright, *Lunacy in India*, p. 12.
[113] Ibid., p. 112.
[114] From Asst. Surgeon J.A. Maxwell to the Chief Secretary to the Government of Bombay, 4 June 1814, GoB, PDD, 1814/368, MSA.
[115] The same as 'Siddi', an ethnic group in India. 'In Pakistan, locals of black African descent are called "Makrani", "Sheedi" or "Habshi". They live primarily along the Makran Coast in Baluchistan, and lower Sindh.' See R. Shekhawat, 'Black Sufis: Preserving the Siddi's and its Age-Old Culture in India', 4th Indian Hospitality Congress, India, Paper Presentation, 2012.
[116] APR, 1873–1874, p. 44, NLS.
[117] APR, 1873–1874, p. 13, NLS.
[118] From the Senior Magistrate of Police to the Secretary to the Government of Bombay, 7 February 1853, GoB, GD, 1853/48, MSA.

two cases of death reported at the Colaba Lunatic Asylum, under the superintendence of Dr. Niven. The first was the death of an Indian patient, Gunoo, who died because of a fractured rib. The Visitors, who made 'enquires among the patients' and the warders, investigated the matter. It was concluded that it was either the 'sane attendants' or the 'insane persons' who had beaten Gunoo. The attendants, however, refused to confess and the Visitors labelled the patients as incompetent witnesses.[119] In another instance in 1871 when a patient committed suicide by hanging, Private Lennon a fellow European inmate was one of the main witnesses in the case. The Coroner who interviewed Private Lennon remarked that he 'was justified in taking the evidence of Private Lennon ... [since] after an examination, I was convinced that he understood the nature of an oath'.[120] When criminal patient Jiva murdered a worker fixing a water pipe at the Ratnagiri Lunatic Asylum in 1912, the superintendent recorded the statements of two Indian patients as witnesses in the case.[121] Asylum staff and other government agencies permitted patients to speak for the purposes of gathering information, but they silenced or selectively heard patients if their information threatened the agency of the asylum staff.

Asylum staff manipulated patients' voices behind asylum walls. Sajan Curim, a Parsi paying patient, complained that when Visitors visited the asylum, 'the stewards, apothecary surgeon, [stood] in front and they ... [did] not allow any complaint to go to them'. Staff physically distanced patients from the Visitors to prevent the hearing of their voices. Subordinate staff even reported the conversations between relatives or friends and patients to their superiors.[122] They also punished patients who made verbal complaints. Miss Shepherd, the Chaplain at Colaba Lunatic Asylum, observed that 'if inmates complained to the Doctors, in any way, the ayahs, they put them in the barred rooms'.[123] In Sajan Curim's case, when he asked warders for water to dilute the *fenny* given to him, he was refused

[119] From the Visitors, Lunatic Asylum, Colaba, to the Secretary to the Government of Bombay, 23 August 1870, JD, GoB, GD, 1870/9, MSA.

[120] From the Coroner of Bombay to the Secretary to the Government, JD, 15 March 1871, GoB, GD, 1871/34, MSA.

[121] Statement of Ganapaya Shankar, Patient in the Lunatic Asylum [Ratnagiri], 14 January 1912, Government of Bombay, General Department, 1912/95, MSA, Mumbai; Statement of Shabas Shiwa Bhajwe, Patient in the Lunatic Asylum [Ratnagiri], 14 January 1912, GoB, GD, 1912/95, MSA.

[122] From Miss Mary Shepherd, W.C.C. Fort, 21 May 1904, GoB, GD, 1904/57, MSA.

[123] From Miss Mary Shepherd, W.C.C. Fort, 21 May 1904, GoB, GD, 1904/57, MSA.

and beaten up. 'No heed was paid' to patients' voices if they requested better conditions.[124]

The control exerted by the asylum staff over patients' voices continued to influence the perception of a patient's sanity even after they left the asylum. Two doctors had certified Sajan Curim as 'perfectly sane' based on his 'coherent conversations'. Three years after the superintendent discharged him from the Colaba Lunatic Asylum, he wrote a letter of complaint to the government. Curim[125] was literate, and his letter proved that he was well versed in lunacy laws. He complained of the mismanagement at the Colaba Lunatic Asylum and the fact that he was not issued a 'Certificate of Admission' even after his release. Curim also brought to light several other problems that patients faced within the asylum.

Hearing patients was an important part of the diagnostic process; however, in the experience of patients, they felt that asylum staff did not hear them. Curim complained of the neglect of the Superintendent, who lived close by but did not pay enough visits to monitor the health of the patients. The Superintendent, he noted, had not issued him a medical certificate. Moreover, he explained that the stewards and apothecary surgeon obstructed patients from complaining to asylum Visitors.[126] Curim further stated that asylum staff forced patients to have cold showers and confined them at regular intervals. A stack of straw served as beds for patients; this, Curim explained, could be 'highly destructive'. He added that the noise of the conversations between asylum staff, especially during the night, disturbed the patients.[127] When patients made requests for any necessities, asylum staff did not pay heed, and at times were even violent towards patients. In an earlier letter, Curim had notified the superintendent that subordinate staff beat him during the night.[128] Curim's letter is clearly coherent and in many ways offered practical suggestions for much needed improvements. Even though he wrote this letter a few years after his discharge, the Superintendent used the letter against Curim.

---

[124] From Sajan Curim to the Superintendent, Lunatic Asylum, Colaba, 17 October 1891, GoB, GD, 1893/75, MSA; From Sajan Curim to the Secretary to the Government of Bombay, 16 October 1893, GoB, GD, 1893/75, MSA.

[125] Curim's letters are the only written sources by an Indian patient for the period of the study (1793–1921). See Appendix 2 for Curim's letters.

[126] From Sajan Curim to the Secretary to the Government of Bombay, 16 October 1893, GoB, GD, 1893/75, MSA.

[127] From Sajan Curim to the Secretary to the Government of Bombay, 16 October 1893, GoB, GD, 1893/75, MSA.

[128] Ibid.

Patients' voices were vulnerable to medical interpretation even years after their discharge from the asylum. In Curim's case, the government enquired into the matter. The Superintendent used Curim's letter as proof of his insanity. In reply to the government, the Superintendent stated that 'from the tenor of the language and the absurd statements in the letter ... he [Sajan Curim] is still suffering from mental troubles'. He went on to interpret Curim's letter as evidence of the 'recurring nature' of his insanity and noted that Curim had had another relapse.[129] In Curim's case, the superintendent wrongly interpreted his voice, manipulated it, and used it against him. Superintendent Keith's interviews with former patients suffering from toxic insanity also provide evidence of control over patients' voices beyond asylum walls. He located former patients and interviewed them regarding their use of hemp. In these cases, superintendents like Dr. Keith manipulated and misinterpreted patients' voices to prove that their entries on patients suffering from hemp insanity were true.[130] Despite such attempts to exert control over patients' voices, there were times when patients' voices reached their local communities.

Once outside the asylum, former patients engaged in slandering the asylum. In 1847, the Assistant Surgeon of the Colaba Lunatic Asylum brought to the notice of the Medical Board that Sepahees who were former patients at the Asylum were spreading word about it. Sepahees or Sipahis were a local Muslim community who were originally from Kathiawar. The *Gazetteer of the Bombay Presidency, Thana*, describes them as a poorer class who indulged in 'opium eating, hemp smoking and palm juice drinking'.[131] The Sepahees were dissuading the local community from using the asylum and instead encouraging them 'to resort for the cure of insanity to idols, incantations and reputed saints, rather than to the asylum'.[132] While patients could not resist asylum agency through force, their slandering of the asylum was a means of resistance.

---

[129] From the Superintendent, Colaba Lunatic Asylum, to the Secretary to the Surgeon General with the Government of Bombay, 5 November 1893, GoB, GD, 1893/75, MSA.

[130] Report of the Indian Hemp Drugs Commission, 1894–1895, Vol. 2, pp. 182–195, NLS.

[131] *Sepahees* or *Sipahis* were a local Muslim community who were originally from Kathiawar. The Gazetteer of Thana describes them as a poorer class who indulged in 'opium eating, hemp smoking and palm juice drinking'. See James Campbell (ed.), *Gazetteer of the Bombay Presidency: Thana*, Vol. XIII (Bombay: Government Central Press, 1882), p. 244.

[132] From the Asst. Surgeon, Colaba Lunatic Asylum, to the Secretary of the Medical Board, 21 February 1847, GoB, GD, 1847/41, MSA.

CONCLUSION

Superintendents and asylum staff failed to achieve sonic hegemony in Bombay's asylums. Bombay's asylum soundscapes were characterized by 'uproar and confusion' compared to the 'regulated and regimented' asylum soundscapes in Britain and her colonies like Australia and New Zealand.[133] Padded cells remained peripheral to noise control in Bombay's asylums. Overcrowding and financial stress posed a substantial challenge to the regulation of sound and noise. Indian languages dominated the aural environment. Occasionally, comforting sounds of music filled the asylum space, interrupting the 'cries of unhappy lunatics'. While asylum agencies permitted patients to 'shout to [their] heart's content', their voices and silences were evaluated, interpreted, and manipulated. Patients' voices were significant because they had both diagnostic and evidential value. Asylum staff interpreted patients' voices within and beyond asylum walls. The manipulation and censoring of these voices protected the asylum staff from coming under government censure. The government ignored the complaints of patients, choosing the narratives of the superintendents over those of the patients. This choice prevented a public scandal and saved government expenditure, but it delayed improvements. The 'cries' heard from within the asylum were evidently 'unhappy'.

In the final chapter, the book moves from within the asylum to its external environment. The next chapter evaluates public perceptions of the asylum. It examines the extent to which the image of the lunatic asylum shaped and determined the local community's attitude towards this institution.

---

[133] Mackinnon, 'Hearing Madness', p. 75.

CHAPTER 6

Public Perceptions of the *Pagal Khana*

The asylum medical class was greatly concerned about the public image of the asylum. In 1852, Dr. W. Campbell, Superintendent of the Colaba Lunatic Asylum, discharged '9 native males before they could be pronounced perfectly convalescent'. He justified his decision by stating:

> Some deference must be paid to the prejudices of those around us ... I feel it is the duty to yield to the desires and demands of friends. To refuse always would expose the institution to the risk of being viewed as a place of captivity where men are incarcerated in defiance of the wishes of those most near and dear to them, rather than a place of cure. It is manifestly of great importance that the native community should have correct notions of the nature and object of the institution.[1]

Dr. Campbell compromised on the regular medical code because in his view, the reputation of the asylum was crucial to its success as a medical institution. Despite the efforts of the medical class to project the asylum as a curative institution, local communities responded with apparent apathy.

The question of the lunatic asylum serving as a curative institution in the Indian colony was a contentious issue. After the British established political hegemony in India, colonial 'Jails, schools and dispensaries'

---

[1] Report on the Lunatic Asylum at Colaba for the Year Ending 1852, GoB, GD, 1853/48, MSA, Mumbai.

© The Author(s) 2018
S. A. Pinto, *Lunatic Asylums in Colonial Bombay,*
Mental Health in Historical Perspective,
https://doi.org/10.1007/978-3-319-94244-5_6

became 'citadels'[2] of British supremacy. Colonial agencies, however, stood divided in their opinion about the lunatic asylum. Only a few medical officers shared Surgeon J. Macpherson's vision of having an 'asylum in every zilla [district]'.[3] In early 1845, the government began deliberations on the need to establish a lunatic asylum in Dharwar. The Superintending Surgeon of Dharwar wrote to the Medical Board objecting to the plan of establishing a lunatic asylum there. He explained:

> [I]t might be well to consider whether it would be expedient or polite to have small number of lunatic asylums scattered all over the country – I must confess that I should look with dread and alarm on such a system. In our own free and happy land, what abuses have not been detected in such receptacles! And how have the enquiries in Parliament within the last thirty or forty years teemed with the discoveries of gross violations of the liberty of the subjects accompanied in most cases by personal cruelty and outrage! If then such practices could exist among Englishmen, what might not be expected from the Asiatic people of this dark benighted land? ... such institutions instead of a blessing, [could] be a curse to the country.[4]

Surgeons debated and probed the establishment of the lunatic asylum on several counts. They questioned its efficacy as a medical institution and the likelihood of it becoming and abusive institution. As the Superintending Surgeon of Dharwar had explained, unless meticulously supervised, colonial asylums would become places of 'gross violations'.[5] The government, however, notwithstanding the lack of consensus among colonial agencies regarding the need for establishing asylums, continued to establish them. By the early twentieth century, 'much chaos'[6] ruled regarding asylum matters, and lunatic asylums remained mere 'lock-ups'.[7]

---

[2] Waltraud Ernst, 'Idioms of Madness and Colonial Boundaries: The Case of the European and "Native" Mentally Ill in Early Nineteenth-Century British India', *Comparative Studies in Society and History*, Vol. 39, No. 01, January 1997, p. 172.

[3] J. MacPherson, Report on Insanity. Royal Commission on the Sanitary State of the Army in India (London; Eyre & Spottswoode for HMSO 1863), Vol. 1.; Bengal Medical Board to Government, 20 October 1847, in Waltraud Ernst, *Mad Tales from the Raj: Colonial Psychiatry in South Asia, 1800–58* (New York: Anthem Press, 2010), p. 49.

[4] From the Superintending Surgeon, Dharwar, to the Secretary to the Medical Board, 15 March 1845, GoB, GD, 1845/43-94, MSA.

[5] Ibid.

[6] From the Superintendent, Colaba Lunatic Asylum, to the Personal Asst. with the Surgeon General, 14 February, 1905, GoB, GD,1905/55, MSA.

[7] From the Surgeon General with the Government of Bombay to the Secretary to the Government of Bombay, 5 November 1904, GoB, GD, 1905/55, MSA.

Dr. Campbell's words sounded prophetic around the early twentieth century. The local community had come to identify the asylum as 'an institution with a repulsive character of insulation, mystery and darkness'.[8] The local community's perception of the asylum was clearly not ill-founded. Superintendent Dr. Jagoe Shaw of the Central Lunatic Asylum at Yerawada, recognizing that the public image of the asylum was hindering its use, attempted to bring about a change in the Indian perception regarding the lunatic asylum.[9] A staunch advocate of western psychiatry, he began promoting the remodelling of Indian asylums on western lines. Dr. Shaw recommended changing the nomenclature of 'Lunatic Asylum' to 'Mental Hospital'[10]—a change he hoped would influence Indian perceptions of the asylum:

> The days when it was considered a visitation of God or a possession by the devil have gone for some time, but the name 'Lunatic Asylum' for the place in India in which persons were imprisoned for the safety of the public, remains, as also, in the public mind, the ideas associated with the name. So vivid are these associated ideas, that it is a common occurrence for persons bringing in a patient, to ask that they may send him certain patent medicines, and surprise is expressed when it is explained that treatment is provided and that the institutions is in fact a hospital. I have also been frequently asked by relatives of incoming patients whether any hospitals for such patients exists in India, and I know that this is a provision for which there is a persistent demand on the part of the more educated classes of India.[11]

Dr. Shaw rightly understood that over the nineteenth and early twentieth centuries, locals had come to perceive the asylum as a mere place of confinement for incurable 'lunatics', rather than a hospital for their treatment. For the local community, the asylum represented a custodial site rather than a curative institution.

Public perceptions have played an important role in the acceptance and social assimilation of institutions. In his research on asylums in Australia and Ireland, Mark Finnane argued that despite being a state institution, 'popular mentality' played an important role in the 'image and use' of the

[8] Report on the Lunatic Asylum at Colaba for the Year Ending 1852, GoB, GD, 1853/48, MSA.

[9] W.S. Jagoe Shaw, 'The Alienist Department of India', *British Journal of Psychiatry*, Vol. 78, April 1932, p. 331.

[10] Ibid., p. 338.

[11] From the Superintendent, Central Lunatic Asylum, Yerawada, to the Surgeon General with the Government of Bombay, 16 July 1920, GoB, GD, 1922/2257B, MSA.

asylum.[12] Historians have attributed the success of the asylum system in colonies like Australasia and Ireland to the fact that families were convinced of 'asylum efficacy' to negotiate familial conflict; they therefore handed over their mentally ill relatives to the asylum.[13] This chapter argues that in India too, local community's perceptions of the asylum influenced its use and disuse. Analysing the response of Bombay's local communities and families to the asylum system from 1850 to 1921, the chapter contends that contrary to the situations in other colonies, a large part of Indian society remained sceptical of the efficacy of the colonial asylum as a place for treatment. In Indian public opinion, the colonial asylum was not a 'hospital' for the cure of 'mental illness'. As the local name *pagal khana* suggested, it was perceived as a mere 'receptacle' for the 'mad'.[14]

The reluctance on the part of the Indian community to admit relatives to the asylums went beyond the 'dread of the loss of caste and the power of superstition'.[15] The community staunchly adhered to the belief that the colonial asylum was a place of permanent confinement for mentally ill people who were unmanageable or dangerous to society. The asylum gained the reputation of being a shelter for poor and destitute lunatics (across caste groups) and a custodial site for 'criminal lunatics'. In spite of having the advantages of a moderate socio-cultural environment and the generous monetary support of the elite class, a very small section of the Indian population admitted their kin or friends to the asylum. This chapter analyses how the asylum figured in the perspectives of three Indian groups: (1) the elite; (2) the local press; and (3) the general masses.

Bombay's Elite: Leaders and Donors

Bombay's local elite began to associate themselves with the asylum only in the latter half of the nineteenth century. Their association with the asylum was due to philanthropic works. The elite included the financial elite—Bombay's

[12] Mark Finnane, 'Asylums, Families and the State', *History Workshop Journal*, No. 20, Autumn 1985, p. 145.

[13] Ibid., p. 135; Catharine Coleborne, *Madness in the Family: Insanity and Institutions in the Australasian Colonial World, 1860–1914* (Basingstoke: Palgrave Macmillan, 2010), p. 3.

[14] *Pagal* meaning 'mad' and *Khana* meaning 'to hold or to contain'. See John Shakespear, *John Shakespear's Dictionary: Urdu- English and English to Urdu* (Lahore: Sang-e-Meel, 2002), pp. 363, 1395.

[15] From the Asst. Surgeon, Colaba Lunatic Asylum, to the Secretary to the Medical Board, 21 February 1847, GoB, GD,1847/41, MSA.

merchant princes—and the political elite—the 'native' chiefs. Among the local communities in Bombay, Parsi businessmen pioneered the philanthropic movement in India in the nineteenth and twentieth centuries. They considered themselves to be 'naturally and by old association the friends of the English merchants and the humble and constant support of the British government'.[16] Other elite groups from various local communities soon imitated their philanthropy. Their economic status helped them establish a link with the asylum, but it also became a cause of their distance from the asylum for treatment purposes, as they perceived the asylum to be a place for the economically underprivileged.

Colonial asylums in Bombay, unlike other asylums in India, received financial support from local donors. The first asylum built using a public donation was the Sir Cowasji Jehangir Lunatic Asylum in Hyderabad (1871). Sir Cowasji Jehangir, a Parsi businessman and one of the 'merchant princes of Bombay',[17] had close ties with the government. The *Punch* called him the 'reverse of Parsi-monious' for a donation he made to the London Fever Hospital. Compared to his other charities, the asylum was one of his 'minor benefactions'.[18] On his return from Sindh, Sir Alexander Grant, Baronet and Director of Public Instruction in the Bombay Presidency, mentioned the need for a lunatic asylum in Sindh. Sir Jehangir promptly made an offer to the government. In 1868, he committed to donating '50,000 Rupees towards a substantially built building and a large garden' in Sindh. He also appealed for 'An assistant surgeon or surgeon of the Government's covenanted service ... [to] be its Superintendent, as now at Bombay ... The Asylum must always be in charge of covenanted doctors under government services'.[19]

Other Indian elite soon emulated Parsi philanthropy. In 1873, local 'chieftains' made a contribution to the Colaba Lunatic Asylum much to the relief of the superintendent. These local chiefs were elite men who assumed leadership of small portions of land, and in some cases even had their own soldiers and collected revenue from the local community. They were descendants of native princes or had held prominent positions under

---

[16] Jehangir Cowasji Jehangir, *Life of Sir Cowasjee Jehangir Readymoney, Kt., C.S.I., &c., &c* (London: London Stereoscopic and Photographic Company, 1890), pp. 7–8.

[17] Dinsha Edulji Wacha, *A Financial Chapter in the History of Bombay City* (Bombay: A.J. Combridge and Co., 1910), p. 202.

[18] Jehangir, *Life of Sir Cowasjee*, p. 23.

[19] Ibid., pp. 52–53.

the Mughal and Maratha rule.[20] The Superintendent at Colaba exclaimed that the Working and Relief fund enjoyed a 'flourishing condition' because of the 'several donations ... from native chiefs'. The chiefs, he added, 'had been led by philanthropic motives and a laudable desire to visit the institution, to gain information about their afflicted countrymen, and observe our mode of treating them'.[21] The following year a 'native Chief', after visiting the asylum, made a personal donation of Rs. 20 to the Superintendent. The Superintendent wrote to the Surgeon General seeking his advice on the matter, since he knew that other native chiefs would follow suite.[22] The asylum became a site for local chiefs to make donations. Superintendents obliged because of the need for funds and it also gave these local leaders a means to associate themselves with the government. The government, however, despised the practice of 'native chiefs' making individual contributions; the superintendent was asked to reject any further donations from native chiefs and the money was to be submitted to the civil treasury.[23] By the latter half of the nineteenth century, Hindu and Muslim elite entered into a 'competitive civic philanthropy' with the Parsis.[24]

Elite Hindu families became associated with local asylums only at the end of the nineteenth century. In 1895, the Madhavdas family contributed Rs. 100,000 towards the building of the new asylum at Naupada, Thana.[25] Furthermore, Seth[26] Narotamdas Madhavdas' widow, Bai Putlibai, left behind a trust fund of Rs. 30,000 which her son Harkishandas Narotamdas

---

[20] There was rivalry among these native chiefs. At times they even collaborated with the British government for political reasons. See James Campbell, *Gazetteer of the Bombay Presidency: Belgaum District* (Bombay: Government Central Press, 1884), pp. 380, 547, 593.

[21] APR, 1873–1874, p. 6, NLS.

[22] From the Superintendent, Lunatic Asylum, Colaba, to the Deputy Surgeon General, IMD, 30 October 1875, GD, 1875/37, MSA.

[23] From the Surgeon General, IMD, to the Secretary to the Government of Bombay, 5 November 1875, GoB, GD, 1875/ 37, MSA.

[24] David Arnold, *Colonizing the Body: State Medicine and Epidemic Disease in Nineteenth-Century India* (Berkley and California: University of California Press, 1993), p. 272.

[25] General Department Compilation 1896, No. 379, (S233), GoB, GD, 1896/81, MSA; PWD, Vol. 533 of 97–99, GoB, GD, 1901/66, MSA. The stone tablet mentions the sum of Rs. 1,15,000: Rs. 86,250 donated by Bai Putlibai and Rs. 28,750 donated by her sons. Marble stone tablet at the Narotamdas Madhavdas Lunatic Asylum (NMLA); see Appendix 1, Fig. A.2.

[26] Seth or Sethia was a title used by 'traditional men of wealth and the rising class of Indian entrepreneurs'. See Shirish Kavadi, 'Philanthropy, Medicine and Health in Colonial India',

assigned for the care of 'pauper high class Hindu lunatics'.[27] Seth Rantansey Premji donated Rs. 12,000 in 1920, for a separate ward for 'better class Hindu lunatics'.[28] The ward provided accommodation for five patients.[29] The practice of philanthropy among Bombay's elite had various connotations.

The asylum for its elite donors was a means of enhancing their own power within colonial society. Douglas Haynes has argued that the 'Gifts and loans ... solidify clientage relations with political overlords.'[30] In the nineteenth century, under colonial rule, the practice of paying tributes changed into the practice of philanthropy.[31] Sir Cowasji Jehangir, in funding the asylum at Hyderabad, made it clear that his donation was made not only for the benefit of his fellow countrymen, but 'with the view of saving so much of the public revenue'.[32] He also added that his contribution would benefit the colonial state, as the asylum building would remain a sign of the lasting legacy of the government:

[The asylum should be] built in modern style, so as to be attractive to the passers-by, who may enquire and finding what it contains may go in and drop some money for the additional comforts of their co-creatures, the lunatics and at the same time for centuries to come such style of buildings will give reflection with high honour to the name of the Englishmen's architecture.[33]

The elite used the asylum as a site for affirming their continued collaboration with the government. The government, in turn, used these local elite agencies as effective 'channels of stabilizing the colonial system'.[34] They

Encyclopaedia of the History of Science, Technology, and Medicine in Colonial India (Netherlands: Springer, 2015), p. 1.

[27] Draft Proposal of the Bai Putlibai Legacy of Rs. 30,000, GoB, GD, 1897/68, MSA.

[28] From Ratansey Premji, Esquire, to the Superintendent, Narotamdas Madhavdas Lunatic Asylum, 12 April 1920, GoB, GD, 1920/1139, MSA.

[29] From Ratansey Premji, Esquire to the Superintendent, Narotamdas Madhavdas Lunatic Asylum, 13 September 1920, GoB, GD, 1920/1139, MSA.

[30] D.E. Haynes, 'From Tribute to Philanthropy: The Politics of Gift Giving in a Western Indian City', *The Journal of Asian Studies*, Vol. 46, No. 2, May 1987, p. 348.

[31] Ibid., pp. 348, 350.

[32] Jehangir, *Life of Sir Cowasjee*, p. 53.

[33] Ibid., p. 54.

[34] Eckeard Kulke, *The Parsees in India: A Minority as Agent of Social Change* (Munchen: Weltforum Verlag, 1974), p. 138.

became bulwarks of the colonial government in India as they aimed at 'securing for the British government in India a feeling of loyalty from other natives'.[35]

Bombay's elite used their philanthropic association with the asylum as a 'path to the attainment of honours from the administration'.[36] Sir Cowasji Jehangir and Narotamdas Madhavdas made donations for the asylums at Hyderabad and Thana on the condition that the government would name the asylums after them. The Madhavdas family also asked for the installation of a marble stone tablet in honour of Narotamdas Madhavdas at the asylum.[37] Sir Cowasji Jehangir made a complaint when the advertisement announcing the opening of the asylum did not refer to it as the Sir Cowasji Jehangir Lunatic Asylum.[38] Bai Dinshaw Petit, widow of the Parsi businessman Nasarvanji Manekji Petit, donated Rs. 15,000 which she later increased to Rs. 20,000 for a separate ward for Parsi patients in the Central Lunatic Asylum at Yerawada. She asked for a 'tablet in a conspicuous place bearing his name'.[39]

Bombay's elite also used the asylum as a space to demonstrate leadership of their own communities. They used their influence to pressurize the government to accommodate the practices, habits, and customs of their respective communities. When the government proposed the construction of a new asylum building at Naupada in 1894, elite Parsis like Sir Dinshaw Manekji Petit and Jamsetji Jejeebhoy led their community in putting together a signature campaign opposing the shifting of the asylum. About 400 members of the Parsi community signed the petition that stated that the chief reasons for opposing the shifting of the asylum were its 'unhealthy location' and 'distance', and 'reluctance to send relatives to such a distance'.[40] The offer of Rs. 20,000 made by the Petit

---

[35] Dosabhoy Framjee, *The Parsees: Their History, Manners, Customs and Religions* (Bombay, London: Smith Elder and Co, 1858), p. 283.

[36] Haynes, 'From Tribute to Philanthropy', p. 351.

[37] From the Executive Engineer to Harkisandas Madhavdas, 24 December 1901, GoB, GD, 1901/61, MSA.

[38] From Sir Cowasji Jehangir to the Secretary to the Government, 21 July 1871, GoB, GD, 1871/34, MSA.

[39] From Dinshaw Master, L.M.&S, Honorary Physician, The Nasarvanji Manekji Petit Charity Fund for Destitute Insane Patients, to the Acting Chief Secretary to the Government of Bombay, 5 February 1894, GoB, GD, 1895/77, MSA.

[40] From Dinshaw Manekji Petit (Signed by the inhabitants) to the Governor and President in Council of the City of Bombay, 10 December 1894, GoB, GD, 1895/77, MSA.

family for two separate wards for male and female Parsis was justified on the grounds that

> Parsi patients, however poor, as a rule, do not like to resort to a hospital where patients of all nationalities are put together in the same ward, and this reluctance is shown not only on religious grounds but also on grounds of cleanliness. The lower classes of natives [who], as a rule, resort to hospitals are very filthy in their habits, and Parsis, as a rule being more cleanly of habits, do not therefore like to associate with them in the same wards.[41]

While asserting leadership of their own community, the Parsis also emphasized their superiority over other Indian communities by distinguishing themselves from the 'natives' and identifying themselves as 'most nearly approximate to Europeans' in habits and customs.[42] The Hindu elite primarily took initiatives to promote religious causes. The Bai Putlibai Trust Fund intended to make provisions in the lunatic asylums for 'ceremonies that every orthodox Hindu performs … worshipping of certain idols and the saying of prayers before them'.[43] The government, however, refused to concede to this demand.[44] While both Parsis and Hindu elite acted to defend and propagate the customs and habits of their communities in the asylum, the Parsi elite used the asylum to assert presumptions of their 'Europeanness' and live the fantasy of assuming leadership of the Indian community.

Bombay's local elite perceived the asylum as an institution for the poor who suffered from mental illness. The patients at the Colaba Lunatic Asylum, as reported by the Assistant Surgeon, were from the 'lowest caste and classes of society'.[45] The Surgeon General of the IMD highlighted the need 'to induce well-off natives to send their relatives to the asylum' in the Annual Asylum Reports for 1874–1875.[46] Parsi patients at Colaba were from the poorer class and the N.M. Petit Parsi Fund set up for destitute Parsis sup-

---

[41] From Dinshaw Master, L.M.&S, Honorary Physician to the Governor in Council, 28 June 1895, GoB, GD, 1900/62, MSA.

[42] Framjee, *The Parsees: Their History, Manners, Customs and Religions*, p. 281.

[43] From Harkisandas Madhavdas to the Secretary to the Government of Bombay, 6 August 1896, GoB, GD, 1896/81 MSA.

[44] From the Secretary to the Govt. to the Surgeon General, Bombay Castle, 12 September 1896, GoB, GD, 1896/81, MSA.

[45] Asst. Surgeon, Colaba Lunatic Asylum, to the Secretary of the Medical Board, 21 February 1847, GoB, GD, 1847/41, MSA.

[46] APR, 1874–1875, p. 15, NLS.

ported their stay at the asylum.[47] The donations from the Madhavdas family were meant for the 'pauper high-class Hindus'.[48] Furthermore, local elite in Bombay refused to send their relatives to the Colaba Lunatic Asylum in spite of it being the 'most expensive' asylum of the Presidency, because they thought 'criminal lunatics' from all over the Presidency were sent there for treatment.[49] For Bombay's influential circle, the asylum was politically significant, but it did not serve them as a curative institution. At the Hyderabad Lunatic Asylum, while 'many respectable natives ... were pleased with the arrangements', they only admitted poor relatives.[50] The elite also perceived the public asylum as lacking in 'scientific treatment'. The elite wanted a private asylum and the lack of it, the *Jam-e-Jamshed* noted, was the reason 'well to do lunatics whose guardians were willing to pay for their treatment, were denied the benefits of professional treatment'.[51]

THE LOCAL PRESS: THE ASYLUM SCANDAL

Miss Mary Shepherd, the Chaplain for the Colaba Lunatic Asylum, was a regular visitor to the patients.[52] On one of her visits in 1904,[53] she described the condition of patients there: 'For months I found in the middle wild beast den – called the "the padded room" – a poor lady without any clothes on! and a Parsee woman in each of the other dens in the same condition!'[54] Appalled by their condition, she threatened Superintendent J. P. Barry with 'the Reporters'. Superintendent Barry immediately responded by refusing her a visiting pass into the asylum since she was 'trying to blacken its character in public opinion'.[55] Superintendent Barry was afraid that 'the Reporters' would tarnish his and the asylum's reputation.

[47] From the Surgeon General to the Secretary to Government, 23 June 1902, GOB, GD, 1902/61, MSA.

[48] Draft Proposal of the Bai Putlibai Legacy of Rs. 30,000, GoB, GD, 1897/68, MSA.

[49] APR, 1874–1875, p. 15, NLS.

[50] Nawab Muhamad Khan, an influential resident of Hyderabad, 'brought a poor relation of his own'. From Superintendent J. Homstead, Cowasjee Jehangir Lunatic Asylum, to the Collector of Hyderabad, 8 July 1874, GoB, GD, 1875/83, MSA.

[51] RNP, *Jam-e-Jamshed*, 20 April 1889, K 416, J–D, PG 1-160, 1889, GoB, MSA..

[52] Miss Mary Shepherd worked as an honorary worker under the Church of England.

[53] By 1904, only Parsi and European patients remained at the Colaba Lunatic Asylum.

[54] From Miss Mary Shepherd to the Governor in Council, 31 May 1904, GoB, GD, 1904/57, MSA.

[55] From Lt. Col. J.P. Barry, Superintendent, Colaba Lunatic Asylum, to J.H. Boulay, 5 June 1904, GD, 1904/57, MSA.

Newspapers and periodicals played an important role in shaping public opinion about colonial rule.[56] The press in colonial Bombay included English, Anglo-Indian, and vernacular newspapers and periodicals. The English press acted with a 'sense of responsibility and under restraint'. The vernacular press in India, however, was more forthright, providing 'valuable moral tales about corruption as well as ... helpful descriptions of the working of many institutions'.[57] The press that the government intended to be the 'handmaiden of Empire' became a cause of great concern as it began criticizing government policies and institutions. The colonial government imposed stringent measures of censorship because of the unease caused by the press. In 1878, the government passed the Vernacular Press Act.[58] It also maintained surveillance by translating abstracts from vernacular newspapers and compiling Native Newspaper Reports to keep a check on 'seditious writing'.[59] This section primarily uses Anglo-Indian and vernacular newspapers and periodicals compiled in the Native Newspaper Reports to construct Indian perceptions of the colonial asylum system in colonial Bombay.

The local press derided the colonial asylum for its lack of 'scientific' treatment. The earliest reference to the asylum in a local newspaper was in 1852. This newspaper reported the state of affairs at the Colaba Lunatic Asylum. Dr. Campbell, who superintended the asylum at the time, addressed the issue in his annual report for the asylum. Highly disapproving of the writer's views, he stated:

> A writer in one of our daily papers, whose favourite term for the Institution of which I have charge is 'The Colaba Abomination' who speaks of its wards and apartments as 'Dungeons' and in the effervescence of a virtuous but somewhat misapplied indignations has not hesitated to stigmatize the treatment to which its inmates are subjected as a 'Disgrace to the British Government and name'.[60]

[56] U. Kalpagam, 'Colonial Governmentality and the Public Sphere in India', *Journal of Historical Sociology*, Vol. 15, No. 1, March 2002, p. 39.

[57] Aakhil Gupta, 'Blurred Boundaries: The Discourse of Corruption, the Culture of Politics, and the Imagined State', *American Ethnologist*, Vol. 22, No. 2, May 1995, pp. 375–402 in Ursula Rao, *News as Culture: Journalistic Practices and the Remaking of Indian Leadership Traditions* (New York: Berghahn Books, 2010), p. 79.

[58] Kalpagam, 'Colonial Governmentality', p. 52.

[59] Ibid., p. 45.

[60] Report on the Lunatic Asylum at Colaba for the Year Ending 1852, GoB, GD, 1853/48, MSA.

Situating the asylum within the larger public debates on public health, the press contended that the government had neglected 'the spread of European medical knowledge and practice in this country'.[61] The *Ahmedabad Samachar* reported: 'The reason [for] so few people going to these institutions [was] that no good medicines … [were] dispensed there … Government itself practice[d] great economy in supplying them with medicines'.[62] The *Indu Prakash,* an Anglo-Marathi newspaper, alleged that the government spent 'millions of money on so-called Public Works Department … [while it did not] pay any attention to the above good work'.[63] The local press presented the asylum as another neglected public health institution of the PWD.

The press also played an important role in exposing the ill-treatment of patients at the asylum. In 1880, a writer in the *Akbari Saudagar* criticized asylum authorities for sending a 'gang of 15–20 patients' under the charge of 'one or two peons', since 'the practice of making patients walk in the intense heat of the summer day, even occasionally is calculated to do injury to their health'. Moreover, he explained, that the Superintendent sent these patients when the streets were 'thronged with people'. He condemned the practice since it could result in 'serious mishaps to the lunatics'.[64] The Native Newspaper Report translated this excerpt from the *Akbari Saudagar* and brought it to the government's notice. Based on this report, the government questioned the Superintendent who admitted to the outdoor labouring of patients. The Superintendent justified his actions to the government by explaining that asylum staff at the Colaba Lunatic Asylum, owing to the lack of space for cultivation, had always made patients undertake outside labour.[65] Apart from objecting to the labouring of patients, the press also advocated for better facilities for them.

In 1880, the *Rast Goftar* staunchly opposed the moving of the Colaba Lunatic Asylum to the Byculla Clubhouse.[66] The Asylum was located at

[61] RNP, *Indu Prakash,* 8 June 1868, GD, K401, J–D, PG 1-424, 1868, GoB, MSA. The *Indu Prakash* was an Anglo-Marathi weekly from Bombay.

[62] RNP, *Ahmedabad Samachar,* 16 October 1878, Week ending 26 October 1878, GoB, MSA.

[63] RNP, *Indu Prakash,* 8 June 1868, GD, K401, J–D, PG 1-424, 1868, GoB, MSA.

[64] RNP, *Akbari Sowdagar,* 13 April 1871, pg. 1-543, GD, K 406, J–D, GoB, MSA.

[65] From the Superintendent, Colaba Lunatic Asylum, to the Deputy Inspector General of Hospitals, IMD, 29 April 1871, GoB, GD, 1871/34, MSA.

[66] Established in 1833, the Byculla Club provided a resting place for Europeans travelling in the *mofussil.* Samuel T. Sheppard, *The Byculla Club, 1833–1916: A History* (Bombay: Bennet, Coleman and Co., 1916), p. 24.

the end of Colaba Island, in close proximity to the Fort or European town. The Club had failed to find a spot closer to the Fort or European town[67] when it was established, and from 1837, the Club committee made attempts to move it to the Fort area. Byculla was 'one of the numerous villages outside the Fort' that was known for its robbers, mosquitoes, and uncovered drains.[68] In 1879, there was a rumour that the government intended to turn the Club into a 'native club or lunatic asylum'.[69] The *Rast Goftar* argued that the location was 'unhealthy on account of it being close to the main drain' and a 'locality which is unhealthy for Europeans cannot but prove equally detrimental to the health of lunatics'.[70] The newspaper also accused the government of corruption, as it alleged that the Club was trying to arrange to get funds in exchange, for building a new clubhouse at the main town near Churchgate station.[71] Along with condemning the mismanagement of asylums, the press also criticized the government for its policy concerning asylum fees.

The local press projected admission to the lunatic asylum as an expensive affair. In 1870, the *Bombay Chabuk* reported that 'if a private person sends mad persons to be lodged, excessive fees are demanded for their admission'.[72] Condemning the authorities for charging high fees, it pleaded that the authorities 'do away with or at least reduce fees at once'.[73] The practice of charging a fee for admission, nevertheless, continued into the twentieth century. The *Bombay Samachar,* a Gujarati weekly, in 1906 reported that 'those who ... [did] not pay a certain initial charge ... [were]

---

[67] The Fort was the 'European town' that developed around Bombay Castle. The Europeans resided in the southern portion, while wealthy Indian merchants occupied the northern portion of the Fort. Meera Kosambi, 'Konkan Ports and European Dominance: An Urban Perspective', in A. R Kulkarni, M.A. Nayeem, T.R. de Souza (eds.), *Mediaeval Deccan History: Commemoration Volume in Honour of Purshottam Mahadeo Joshi* (Bombay: Popular Prakashan, 1996), p. 119.

[68] Sheppard, *The Byculla Club,* pp. 1, 46.

[69] Ibid., pp. 47–48.

[70] RNP, *Rast Goftar,* 9 May 1880, GD, K-409I, J–D, PG 1-444, 1880, GoB, MSA. The *Rast Goftar* was a Gujarati Weekly from Bombay.

[71] RNP, *Rast Goftar,* 9 May 1880, GD, K-409I, J–D, PG 1-444, 1880, GoB, MSA.

[72] RNP, *Bombay Chabuk,* 13 July 1870, GD, K404/ 251, J–D, PG 1-543, GoB, MSA. The *Bombay Chabuk* was a Gujarati weekly. For 'natives', asylum rates were as follows: first class patients Rs. 2, second class patients Rs. 1, third class patients 8 annas and fourth class patients 4 annas. (An anna to a rupee is like a penny to a dollar). Government Resolution (GR), General Department, 12 November 1874, No. 3247, GoB, GD, 1916/111, MSA.

[73] RNP, *Bombay Chabuk,* 13 July 1870, GD, K404/ 251, J–D, PG 1-543, GoB, MSA.

refused admission into the asylum'. The newspaper petitioned for a change and stated that 'were it not for the apathy of the native community in taking advantage of these institutions, this grievance would be regarded as a public scandal'.[74] The government refused to address the grievances of the press. Rather, by 1915, even non-paying patients who were not 'well to do' had to pay for food. Only 'destitute patients' were given free food from the hospital or dispensary.[75] While making complaints about the asylum system, the press also made suggestions to the government for improvements to it.

The press made recommendations to the state and petitioned Bombay's local elite to collaborate and work towards a solution to the asylum scandal. The *Jam-e-Jamshed,* referring to the Asylum Reports for the year 1888, pointed out the 'urgent necessity of having a first-class asylum in Bombay'.[76] One newspaper urged the government to 'enlarge the accommodation in existing asylums and to allot larger grants for their proper maintenance'. It also persuaded Indian 'medical men … [to] start private asylums, with the aid of public charity … to supplement the efforts of the government to alleviate the lot of these unfortunate creatures'.[77] The *Nyaya Sindhi,* a Marathi newspaper, opined that the funds raised to commemorate the achievements of Lord Mayo should be used to 'start two to three good asylums for the blind, lame and helpless people'.[78] Vernacular newspapers thus tried to implore the government to pay attention to the improvement of the asylum system.

Vernacular newspapers in India during the nineteenth and early twentieth centuries focused on the twin themes of the 'exploitative character of the colonial state and its indifference to the welfare of the people'.[79] The asylum system, however, was not a major point of discussion; the press directed attention to it only occasionally. In the Bombay Presidency, vernacular newspapers exposed the 'exploitative character' of the asylum

[74] RNP, *Bombay Samachar,* 5 June 1906, GD, J–J, Week ending 9 June 1906, GoB, MSA. The *Bombay Samachar* was a daily newspaper from Bombay.

[75] Rules Governing the Levy of Fees in Government and State Aided Hospitals and Dispensaries (including the city of Bombay and Aden), 24 November 1915, GoB, GD, 1916/111, MSA.

[76] RNP, *Jam-e-Jamshed,* 20 April 1889, GD, K 416, J–D, PG 1-160, 1889, GoB, MSA.

[77] RNP, *Bombay Samachar,* 5 June 1906, GD, J–J, Week ending 9 June 1906, GoB, MSA.

[78] RNP *Nyaya Sindhi,* 20 April 1872, GD, K406, J–D, PG 1-534, GoB, MSA. The *Nyaya Sindhi* was a weekly newspaper from Ahmednagar.

[79] Kalpagam, 'Colonial Governmentality', p. 45.

system on one hand, and on the other, criticized the government for its 'indifference' towards the system that seemingly amounted to a public scandal. The government's mismanagement of lunacy administration continued despite the criticism from the local press. This management caused Indian communities to keep their distance from the asylum. Vernacular newspapers 'instigated a feeling of overt hostility' towards the asylum system and lunacy administration, and therefore had 'a harmful effect on the relations between the government and the people'.[80]

The vernacular press shaped public discourse on the asylum by 'generating critical opinion on governmental action and inaction'.[81] While asylums were peripheral to the public discourse, newspapers kept the asylum and the condition of lunacy administration alive in public memory. The press pictured the asylum as an institution where 'treatment' was costly, and where doctors laboured patients under the pretext of curing their mental illness. The local press thus unintentionally dissuaded people from using the asylum by projecting it as a place that lacked scientific and medical methods of treatment. News of the asylum reached the local masses and kept them away from the *pagal khana*.

THE GENERAL MASSES AND THE ASYLUM

The lunatic asylum left a strong impression on the Indian public mind. Locals popularly called one of the roads leading to the Colaba Lunatic Asylum the 'Asylum Road'. The government had originally named this road Beach Road. It extended from Colaba Road through Back Bay and connected to the gate of the old Lunatic Asylum. The association of the asylum with the road in the public mind was so strong that even after the government closed the Colaba Lunatic Asylum and moved its patients to the new Yerawada Lunatic Asylum in 1914, locals continued to call the road the 'Asylum Road'. After its closure, military authorities insisted that the road be renamed 'Roberts Road', since there was no need 'for maintaining the memory of the Lunatic Asylum'.[82] The renaming was a conscious effort on the part of the government to erase from public memory the association between the street and the asylum that had brought much criticism to it.

---

[80] Ibid., p. 52.
[81] Ibid., p. 44.
[82] Samuel Shephard, *Bombay Place-Names and Street-Names: An Excursion into the By-Ways of the History of Bombay City* (Bombay: Times Press, 1917), p. 126.

The road to the asylum was one that few local families willingly chose to tread. Most patients confined in the asylum were 'wanderers with no friends'.[83] The *Medical Jurisprudence for India* noted that 'voluntary consignment of troublesome lunatics to public asylums [was a] rare occurrence'.[84] Persons who were admitted were usually 'found committing mischief in the public streets and caught and conveyed there by the police'.[85] The families who admitted their relatives or friends did so as a last resort, to confine those who were extremely violent or unmanageable. Julie Parle in her research on Asylums in Zululand argued that '[i]nformal family and social networks remained the first port of call' for locals. Using Leslie Swartz's categorization of mental health and strategies she elaborated that local communities in Africa had three 'sectors' of treatment: the 'professional sector' (mental hospitals and western psychiatry), the 'popular sector' (self-help groups and the like), and the 'folk sector'.[86] The folk sector that included 'African indigenous and faith healers' remained the sector that Africans largely depended on for alleviating mental suffering.[87] These findings also apply to the Indian context. When Indian families failed to manage mental illness within the family, they sought help from the 'folk sector' of traditional healers and caretakers.[88] This section argues that for local families the asylum was merely a receptacle for mentally ill people who had become unmanageable at home or those deemed dangerous to society, rather than a hospital for treating mental illness. Moreover, the asylum failed to provide families any permanent relief from mentally ill relatives, since the colonial state refused to maintain incurable 'lunatics' in the asylum on grounds that they were an additional burden to the state.[89]

---

[83] Report of the Indian Hemp Drugs Commission, 1894–1895, Vol. 1, p. 231, NLS.

[84] Lyon Isidore Bernadotte, *Medical Jurisprudence for India, with Illustrative Cases,* Vol. 7(Calcutta: Thacker and Spink, 1921), p. 329.

[85] RNP, *Bombay Chabuk,* 13 July 1870, GD, K404/ 251, J–D, PG 1-543, GoB, MSA.

[86] Julie Parle, 'Witchcraft or Madness? The Amandiki of Zululand, 1894–1914', *Journal of Southern African Studies,* Vol 29, No. 1, March 2003, pp. 110, 117.

[87] Ibid; Julie Parle, 'States of Mind: Mental illness and the quest for mental health in Natal and Zululand, 1868–1918', PhD Thesis, University of KwaZulu-Natal, 2004, p. viii.

[88] As elaborated in Chap. 2.

[89] 'The inspector must now be informed that harmless and incurable lunatics should not be incarcerated.' From the Director General, IMD (forwarded with remarks), by the Inspector General of Prisons to the Governor in Council, 9 December 1858, GoB, GD, 1859/24, MSA.

The Asylum and Vagrancy Management

Asylum Population Tables included in the Annual Asylum Reports provide important insights into the background of local patients. In these tables, doctors categorized their patients based on district/region, religion, and sex. These tables also incorporated 'caste' as a category. However, doctors used the word 'caste' in a rather fluid manner. The tables fail to mention any actual Indian caste groups. Asylum doctors used the word 'caste' instead of the term 'other religions' or 'race'. 'Caste' groups listed included 'Europeans', 'Eurasians', 'Native Christians', 'Hindoos', 'Muslims', 'Parsees', 'Jews', 'Other castes', and 'occupation'.[90] In terms of actual Indian caste groups, patients came from across such groups. In 1893, as part of the Hemp Commission Report, the government asked superintendents to make inquiries about their patients' histories to ascertain the links between hemp use and insanity. The interviews revealed that patients came from varying caste groups. However, a majority came from 'poorer classes'[91] and were 'wanderers with no friends'.[92]

Beggars, *fakirs*, and mendicants accounted for more than 70 per cent of asylum population in the Presidency.[93] Most of these patients found themselves in an asylum when the police arrested them for 'committing mischief in the public streets'.[94]

The colonial lunatic asylum helped manage indigenous vagrancy. Medieval Indian society 'tolerated' vagrants, beggars, and religious mendicants.[95] The advancement of industrial capitalism, however, created an increasing colonial concern for making local populations productive. Asylums facilitated the internalization of self-discipline to create productive individuals within a society organized on such ideals.[96] In Ahmedabad, the Gazetteer reported that a 'crowd of idlers and beggars' who took a handful of cotton from the bales in the name of 'custom or charity' had 'threated the prosperity of the

[90] APR, 1873–1874, p. 2, NLS; APR, 1904, p. 5, NLS; Triennial Report on the Lunatic Asylums under the Government of Bombay, 1903–1905, p. 9, NLS.

[91] Asst. Surgeon, Colaba Lunatic Asylum to the Secretary of the Medical Board, 21 February 1847, GoB, GD, 1847/41, MSA.

[92] Report of the Indian Hemp Drugs Commission, 1894–1895, Vol. 1, p. 231, NLS.

[93] APR, 1880, p. 2, NLS.

[94] RNP, *Bombay Chabuk*, 13 July 1870, GD, K404/ 251, J–D, PG 1-543, GoB, MSA.

[95] Avishek Ray, 'Archaeology of Vagabondage: South Asia's Colonial Encounter', PhD Thesis, Trent University, 2014, p. ii.

[96] Andrew Scull, *Museums of Madness: The Social Organization of Insanity in Nineteenth-Century England* (London: Trinity Press, 1979), pp. 15, 48, p. 113.

port'.[97] While colonial agencies showed a keen interest in managing vagrancy, it was colonial rule itself that had led to an increase in the number of beggars. Colonial economic exploitation and the Industrial Revolution left indigenous artisans without an income.[98] The official Gazetteers of the Bombay Presidency recorded the increasing number of vagrants across religion, caste, and occupation groups. The Gazetteer for Poona, recorded 23 classes (caste) of Hindu beggars like *A'rádhis* ('praying beggars'), *Bhámtas-* (wandering beggars who chanted), *Bháts* ('hereditary beggars'), and *Ghondalis* (performers of the *ghondal* dance who begged), among many others. The Gazetteer even included *vaids* or physicians as beggars and explained that the 'dispensaries ... and growing trust in English drugs, have ruined the Vaidus' who were now 'little better than beggars'.[99] The government tried to manage vagrancy by passing legislations and establishing institutions.

In 1874, following the passing of the Vagrancy Act, the government established workhouses in Bombay. The government intended these workhouses for European vagrants. Harald Fischer-Tiné argued that these workhouses served the 'internal civilizing mission'. In 1911, when officials observed an increase in 'black inmates' in the Bombay workhouse, they issued a circular excluding Eurasians and Indians from the provisions of the Vagrancy Act. The exclusion of indigenous vagrants from workhouses indicated the colonial concern for maintaining boundaries and hierarchies with the colonial order.[100]

Since workhouses excluded indigenous vagrants, the only other institution that would instil a sense of self-discipline and make vagrants productive was the lunatic asylum. The increasing patient populations of beggars, *fakirs*, and mendicants indicate that the asylums, then, served the government well in managing the increasing indigenous vagrant population. In cases of vagrancy, as discussed earlier, the police initiated the admission process. Local families, however, sought the 'professional sector'[101] of the asylum only when their relatives became unmanageable.

[97] Campbell, James (ed.), *Gazetteer of the Bombay Presidency: Ahmedabad*, Vol. IV (Bombay: Government Central Press, 1879), p. 104.

[98] Dyutimoy Mukherjee, 'Laws for Beggars, Justice for Whom: A Critical Review of the Bombay Prevention of Begging Act 1959', *The International Journal of Human Rights*, Vol. 12, No. 2, April 2008, pp. 280–281.

[99] James Campbell (ed.), *Gazetteers of the Bombay Presidency: Poona*, Vol, XVIII, Part 1 (Bombay: Government Central Press, 1885), pp. 477–479.

[100] Harald Fischer-Tiné, 'Britain's Other Civilizing Mission: Class Prejudice, European 'loaferism' and the Workhouse-system in Colonial India', *The Indian Economic and Social History Review*, Vol. 42, No. 3, 2005, pp. 316–317, 329–330.

[101] Parle, 'Witchcraft or Madness', p. 110.

The Asylum as a Custodial Site for the 'Publicly Dangerous'

In colonial Bombay, the asylum system, the penal system, and the judicial system were intrinsically linked. The common colonial notion was that the 'general tendency of all mental disorders [was] to disturb the balance of the social environment, [and that] it frequently expresse[d] itself in the form of crime'.[102] Even before the Lunacy Act of 1858 legalized the involvement of magistrates in the admission process, the magistrates authoritatively played a role in the committal process. In 1849, Magistrate Bettington committed Brahmin Devram to the asylum for his ritual fasting, since the magistrate believed the Brahmin was attempting suicide. Moreover, the Brahmin, he explained, was 'not judicially cured till he ... [ate] food voluntarily'.[103] Assistant Surgeon Gillanders challenged Magistarte Bettington's diagnosis. Brahmin Devram, nevertheless, remained in the asylum for a few more months until the government sorted out the dispute between the two. As discussed in Chap. 3 of this book, power contestations characterized the relations between the medical and judicial departments. The Lunacy Act of 1858 reinforced the authority of the penal and judicial departments in the committal process. Clause IV of the Act stated that the '*Darogah* or District Police Officer could apprehend or send to magistrates all persons found wandering at large within his district who are deemed to be lunatics and all persons believed to be dangerous by reason of lunacy'.[104] The Lunacy Act gave police the authority to incarcerate and bring before a magistrate persons whom they perceived as suffering from lunacy.

The intrinsic association with the penal and judicial system is also evident from the asylum admission process. The police or families had to present the following before the magistrate for asylum admission:

1. The lunatic
2. Form of Application
3. Two medical certificates, Form 3 (one must be given by a gazetted officer) [This form mentioned the 'Facts indicating insanity']
4. The answer of the superintendent of the asylum.[105] [A letter from the superintendent of accepting the patient in the asylum]

[102] Bernadotte, *Medical Jurisprudence for India*, p. 329.
[103] From the Magistrate of Ahmedabad to the Civil Surgeon, Ahmedabad, 13 August 1849, JD, GoB, GD, 1849/38, MSA.
[104] Lunacy Act XXXVI of 1858, GoB, GD, 1862-64/15, MSA.
[105] Bernadotte, *Medical Jurisprudence for India*, pp. 406–407.

Following an inquiry, the Magistrate would then issue an 'Order for Reception'. Furthermore, the admission process added to the pillory, as magistrates were 'in a habit of holding the inquiry in open court to the great confusion and humiliation of the relations'.[106] By contrast, in Ireland, it was the dissociation of the asylum from criminality and the laws that supported it that helped asylums to achieve legitimacy.[107] The intrinsic links between the asylum and the judicial and penal systems in India, reinforced by the law, added to the stigmatization of the person admitted and their families.

In India, local communities feared the stigma associated with incarceration of their mentally ill relatives by the police. The association of the asylum with the penal and judicial system reinforced the practice of families confining such relatives in their homes, to avoid surveillance and incarceration by the police and magistrates. Dr. Jagoe Shaw, having worked in asylums all over India, elaborated that among the public 'there [existed] a fear of asylums due to the idea that once a person is considered "mad" he must be taken by the police, and shut up for the rest of his life in an asylum'.[108] Even in the early decades of the twentieth century, the local community had the 'common conception' that the lunatic asylum was a 'prison for lunatics'. This conception led to families avoiding the asylum and missing early preventive treatment.[109] In 1915, Chhotalal Sukhadia from Broach applied to the Deputy Collector and Magistrate for the admission of his wife who was a 'lunatic for some past years'. He offered to pay for her treatment at the asylum. The Collector initiated proceedings, making sure that 'special precautions were taken to avoid publicity or anything that could offend the susceptibilities of Chhotalal or his caste'. However, the Collector reported that Chhotalal appealed to him to stop the proceedings because of 'his strong fears of humiliation in the eyes of his caste fellows, due to the police taking action in this case'.[110] In another case, the father of a patient named Dholu explained that 'for two to three months after his release from the asylum, [his son] did not go out of the

---

[106] Ibid., p. 407.

[107] Finnane, 'Asylums, Family and the State', p. 143.

[108] From the Superintendent, Central Lunatic Asylum, Yerawada, to Surgeon General with the Government of Bombay, 16 July 1920, GoB, GD, 1922/2257B, MSA.

[109] From the Superintendent, Central Lunatic Asylum, Yerawada, to Surgeon General with the Government of Bombay, 16 July 1920, GoB, GD, 1922/2257B, MSA.

[110] From the Collector of Broach to the Government of Bombay, 26 April 1915, GoB, GD, 1915/250, MSA.

house through shame'.[111] The fear and stigma experienced by families because of the involvement of the penal and judicial agencies prevented them from using the asylum.

For Indian families, the notion of 'dangerous to the public' had a different meaning that did not go well with the one favoured by the colonial agencies. Families kept internal familial conflicts within the family. Even when the mentally ill person was violent towards family members, families did not commit him/her to an asylum. Relatives only handed over a person who was unmanageable. Superintendent J. Keith of the Hyderabad Lunatic Asylum interviewed Waliram, the father of patient Mulchand, as part of the Hemp Commission Report. He noted that Waliram ascribed his son's insanity to sunstroke he had suffered 10 years prior. Waliram stated that his son 'became gradually insane, and was getting troublesome … he was not dangerous to society, nor did he beat anyone. He, however, used to beat me and his mother sometimes when excited'. Waliram's description suggests his surprise and confusion about his son's asylum confinement since 'he was not dangerous to society',[112] in spite of the history of domestic violence. In the case of another patient, Metho, his family continued to look after him even though he was violent and used abusive language. Indian families did not consider the asylum to be an 'arbiter of family relationships'.[113] They therefore interpreted attempts by police or magistrates to incarcerate an individual as unnecessary acts of forced intervention in private lives.

Through petitions, family members contested forced interventions and admissions. Both close relations and extended family members made petitions for the release of patients from the asylum. Some examples of petitions for the release of immediate family members can be gleaned from cases like that of Dayaram, a resident of Baroda who petitioned for the release of his son Damodar. The District Magistrate of Khandesh committed Damodar to the Colaba Lunatic Asylum.[114] His family was not involved in his admission and it is likely that when the family found out his whereabouts, they applied for his release. In another case in 1897, Bausilal Ramchandra petitioned the government for the release of his relative

[111] Report of the Indian Hemp Drugs Commission, 1894–1895, Vol. 2, p. 184, NLS.
[112] Report of the Indian Hemp Drugs Commission, 1894–1895, Vol. 2, p. 189, NLS.
[113] Finnane, 'Asylums, Family and the State', p. 143; Coleman, *Madness in the Family*, p. 120.
[114] GR, JD, Bombay Castle, 21 February 1901, GoB, GD, 1901/65, MSA.

Vithal Akaji Bari, a patient at the Poona Lunatic Asylum, admitted there for three years. Bausilal claimed that Vithal's condition was 'getting worst and worst gradually'. If the authorities kept him there any longer, he thought, he would 'breathe his last there'. Bausilal promised to stand as a guarantor for Vithal.[115] The asylum and judicial agencies rejected his petition; they released Vithal only in 1899, two years after his relative made the petition.[116] Even when the magistrate had certified a patient as a 'criminal lunatic', his/her family petitioned for their release from the asylum. Table 6.1 lists the numerous petition requests from families for the period 1897–1915. The Table shows that the stigma of incarceration in the asylum was so strong that even families of 'criminal patients' were petitioning for their release. The practice of petitioning for release of relatives became more popular towards the end of the nineteenth and the early decades of the twentieth century, indicating that Indian families increasingly distrusted the efficacy of the asylum system.[117]

When pressured due to financial constraints or unmanageability of patients, Indian families appealed for a transfer, instead of release from the asylum. Sakinabai, from Poona, appealed for the transfer of her son S.K. Kasam. She wrote:

> I beg to state that my son S K Kasam … has no improvement there from the date of admission. I am a poor old woman … I have not seen him in the last six months on account of no money with me. I heard that there are places here in Poona Lunatic Asylum. I hope your honor will transfer him here that I may see him daily here and satisfy my heart … .[118]

Families ensured that their relatives were in an asylum close enough for them to visit frequently, in spite of them being poor. In 1915, Pandu Ram Mochi requested the transfer of his son Ganpat from the Dharwar Lunatic Asylum to the Narotamdas Madhavdas Lunatic Asylum, citing his poverty as a reason for his inability to travel to Dharwar.[119] Superintendents did

[115] From Bausilal Ramchandra to the Under Secretary to the GoB, Poona, 22 February 1897, GD, 1897/68, MSA.

[116] GR, JD, Bombay Castle, 4 July 1899, GoB, GD, 1899/64, MSA.

[117] See Table 6.1.

[118] From Sakinabai to the Superintendent of the Lunatic Asylum, Ahmedabad, 29 December 1909, Poona, GoB, GD, 1909/69, MSA.

[119] From Pandu Ram Mochi to the Personal Asst. to the Surgeon General with the Government of Bombay, Poona, 11 March 1915, GoB, GD, 1915/336, MSA.

Table 6.1 Index of patients whose relatives applied for their discharge, Bombay Presidency (1897–1915)

Year	Petitioner/ guarantee	Relation to patient	Patient	Asylum	Criminal lunatic	Released Yes/ No
1897	Bansilal Ramchandra	Friend	Vithal Akoji Bari	Poona LA	No	No. (released two years later)
1901	Dayaram Jagjivan	Father	Damodar	Colaba LA	No	Yes
1901	Rudrappa	Father	Virbhadrappa	Dharwar LA	No	Yes
1903	Jairam Poma	Cousin	Govind Poma	Ratnagiri LA	No	Yes
1903		Father	Abdul Karim Jusab	NMLA, Thana	Yes (Theft)	Yes
1903		Nephew	Dhondi Anyanbai	NMLA, Thana	Yes (Theft)	Yes
1903	Bai Khatija	Wife	Shek Esuf	Colaba LA	No	No
1903	Kurvabai	Wife	Hormasji Bhatporia	Colaba LA	No	No
1903	Adiveppa Kenchappa	Brother	Bashya Kenchappa	Dharwar LA	Yes	Yes
1909	Jiva Gagal	Brother	Lalu	NMLA, Thana	No	Yes
1909	Moreshwar Divekar	Father	Dhondu Divekar	Ratnagiri LA	Yes (Theft)	Yes
1909		Brother-in-law	Vishnu Purohit	Ratnagiri LA	Yes (Theft)	Yes
1909	Saibai Sonar	Sister	Babu Sitaram Sonar	NMLA, Thana	Yes	Yes
1909	Babu Balu	Brother	Govind Baloba Sutar	NMLA, Thana	Yes (Theft)	Yes
1910	Nadirsha Bagli	Brother	Kavasji Naoroji	Colaba LA	Yes	Yes
1911	Bhanji Ladha	Brother-in-law	Shivji Akhai	NMLA, Thana	No	Yes
1911	Pandu Ram Mochi	Son	Ganpat Pandu	NMLA, Thana	Yes	Yes
1911		Mother	Shankar Ghangale	Poona LA	Yes	Yes
1912		Brother	Shivram Shaligram	Ratnagiri LA	Yes	Yes

(*continued*)

Table 6.1 (continued)

Year	Petitioner/ guarantee	Relation to patient	Patient	Asylum	Criminal lunatic	Released Yes/ No
1912	Gajanan Kulkarni	Brother	Ramchandra Kulkarni	NMLA, Thana	Yes (Theft)	Yes
1913	Narayan Damji	Father	Karuna Shankar	NMLA, Thana	Yes	Yes
1915	Duri	Brother	Afzal Mohammad	Central LA, Yerawada	Yes	No. transferred to CJLA, Hyderabad

Source: Compiled from various files in GoB, GD, MSA
CJLA Sir Cowasji Jehangir lunatic asylum, *LA* lunatic asylum

not like these frequent visits from family members or friends; as one super-intendent complained: 'In comparatively few instances, can natives be made to understand why they should not see persons under treatment, to whom they are allied by the ties of kindred or acquaintanceship'.[120] Andrew Scull, Michel Foucault, and David Wright have argued that the transfor-mation of society on market principles changed Victorian family values and popularized the use of asylums in Britain.[121] By contrast, the petitions of families with patients in the asylums of Bombay reflected the community-centric ideals of Indians.

Superintendents deemed the close family and community ties as obstructions to the healing process of patients. In colonies like New Zealand, contact between families and patients were believed to aid recu-peration of patients.[122] In Bombay, however, doctors deemed it harmful to the treatment process, since 'the great advantage' of asylum admission was 'the separating [of patients] from not only places and things but also from individuals who may be connected with his delusions'. Any interaction with friends and near relatives was therefore considered to be 'extremely

[120] Report on the Lunatic Asylum at Colaba for the Year Ending 1852, GoB, GD, 1853/48, MSA.
[121] Andrew T. Scull, *Museums of Madness: The Social Organization of Insanity in Nineteenth-Century England* (London: Trinity Press, 1979), pp. 15, 48; Michel Foucault, *Madness and Civilization: A History of Insanity in the Age of Reason*, trans. Richard Howard (New York: Vintage Books, 2003) Foucault, pp. 253–256; David Wright, 'Getting Out of the Asylum: Understanding the Confinement of the Insane in the Nineteenth Century', *Social History of Medicine*, Vol. 10, No. 1, 1997, p. 155.
[122] Coleborne, *Madness in the Family*, p. 52.

dangerous'.[123] In the perception of the Indian families, the colonial asylum therefore appeared as a dispensable institution for the care of their relatives who suffered from mental illness. The 'ideal of family responsibility'[124] affected the use of and shaped the attitudes of the Indian people towards the asylum.

The 'ideal of family responsibility' also had a significant impact on the admission of women to the asylum. The *Medical Jurisprudence of India* highlighted the fact, stating: 'A majority of the cases in Indian asylums were males'.[125] In Triennial Reports for Asylums in the Presidency for 1903–1905, Asylum male: female numbers stood as follows: Ratnagiri 10:6, Poona 57:12, Dharwar 12:8, Ahmedabad 16:4, Hyderabad 271:46.[126] Even by 1921, there was little change in admission numbers of local women. In 1921, the numbers stood as follows: Naupada 135:25, Ratnagiri 35:7, Dharwar 30:22, Yerawada 131:16, Ahmedabad 37:20, Hyderabad 572:88.[127] Since doctors in Victorian Britain considered madness as a 'Female Malady', the disparity between admission numbers of men and women drew questions from colonial agencies.[128] The asylum medical staff reported that the 'lower classes' were more willing to admit their females.[129] In 1852, Dr. Campbell also reported that most of the women were from the 'low caste'.[130] In the Asylum Report for 1873, the disparity was blamed on the 'custom of the country to keep women within their own houses' and a general hesitance 'to seek indoor hospital relief' for them. Furthermore, it reiterated that 'unless either very poor or very troublesome their friends seldom seek to have them removed to a lunatic

[123] Report on the Lunatic Asylum at Colaba for the Year Ending 1852, GoB, GD, 1853/48, MSA.

[124] Margaret Tennant argued that in New Zealand the 'ideal of family responsibility … provided a hurdle over which women in particular, might be required to leap before public assistance was forthcoming'. See Margaret Tennant, *Paupers and Providers: Charitable Aid in New Zealand* (Wellington: Allen and Unwin/Historical Branch, 1989), pp. 13–14.

[125] Bernadotte, *Medical Jurisprudence for India*, p. 331.

[126] Triennial Report on the Lunatic Asylums under the Government of Bombay, 1903–1905, pp. 7–8, NLS.

[127] APR, 1921, p. 7, NLS.

[128] Elaine Showalter, *The Female Malady* (New York: Pantheon Books, 1985), p. 7.

[129] From the Asst. Surgeon, Colaba Lunatic Asylum, to the Secretary of the Medical Board, 21 February 1847, GoB, GD, 1847/41, MSA.

[130] Report on the Lunatic Asylum at Colaba for the Year Ending 1852, GoB, GD, 1853/48, MSA.

asylum, but try to manage them at home quietly'.[131] Thus, as David Arnold has argued, their 'elusiveness was an implicit challenge to the hegemonic ambitions of western medicine'.[132]

Culturally insensitive processes connected to the asylum also contributed to the refusal of families to admit their mentally ill women. David Arnold argued that women's general health 'rapidly assumed a remarkable and emblematic position' after the 1870s.[133] The government, however, largely neglected mental health measures for women. *The Medical Jurisprudence* noted that it was the possibility of public exposure that kept Indian families from admitting their women, since Magistrates conducted the process in public places and it 'frequently [led to] painful exhibitions on the part of female lunatics before a ribald audience'.[134] Some of Bombay's asylums were so crowded that staff could not maintain segregation between male and female patients due to spatial constraints.[135] Indian society during this period particularly adhered to the 'exclusion and seclusion'[136] of women, and the lack of segregation was a reason to evade the asylum. Furthermore, asylums in Bombay had no females on the list of government asylum Visitors until the early decades of the twentieth century.[137] Women had no representation for their grievances and no voice behind asylum walls.

The Asylum as a Receptacle for 'Unmanageable' Mentally Ill Persons

Families in colonial Bombay used the asylum only as a last alternative to manage their incurable unmanageable mentally ill relatives. Describing the trend of asylum admission among Indian families in 1844, the Civil Surgeon at Dharwar pointed out that 'the disease is generally allowed to run its course beyond the power of cure before they [the families] will

---

[131] APR, 1873–1874, p. 16, NLS.

[132] Arnold, *Colonizing the Body*, p. 256.

[133] Ibid., p. 54.

[134] Bernadotte, *Medical Jurisprudence for India*, p. 407.

[135] From F.S. Arnott, Inspector General of Hospitals to the Adjutant General of the Army, 12 January 1869, GoB, GD, 1869/4, MSA.

[136] Samita Sen, *Women and Labour in Late Colonial India: The Bengal Jute Industry* (Cambridge: Cambridge University Press, 1999), pp. 60–61.

[137] From Miss Mary Shepherd to the Governor in Council, 31 May 1904, GoB, GD, 1904/57, MSA.

concede to such a separation'.[138] At the Colaba Lunatic Asylum, patients who were admitted had 'passed through the acute forms of the disease which are most curable and [were] rapidly passing into, if they have not already reached the most incurable forms of the disease those of Imbecile and Idiocy'.[139] At the asylum, doctors diagnosed Metho as suffering from 'Toxic Insanity' caused by *ganja* smoking.[140] His family members and acquaintances stated that they admitted him on the recommendation of the Civil Surgeon as a last resort. Oodernomal, his elder brother recounted that Metho left his job and came to live in his house:

> [T]here he showed symptoms of insanity. Was very abusive; used to talk nonsense; ate like a glutton; committed mischief; became violent and troublesome. I then placed him under the treatment of the native *hakim* (quack),[141] but it did him no good. I then took him to the civil hospital, but there too no good was done … I put him under the treatment of Dr Tarachand for a month, but finding no change, I sent him to the Asylum through the Sub-divisional Magistrate … .[142]

Metho was kept in the asylum for a year after which he was sent home, but soon after he 'showed signs of insanity and was worse than before'. Metho's other brother Durrian stated that the second time the family was 'obliged to hand him over to the police who sent him to the Civil Surgeon and then again to the asylum'.[143]

Methos' family denied that he used hemp. However, Superintendent J. Keith, suspicious of the statement made by the family, 'tried an experiment'. He asked a cured patient, Sarandas, to act as a host and offer Metho '*bhang, ganja and charas*'.[144] He reported that Metho was 'most eager … to help in their preparation and to assist in their consumption'. Moreover, he stated that Metho confessed having *bhang, ganja,* and *charas* every day

---

[138] From the Civil Surgeon, Dharwar, to the Commissioner of Bombay, 3 August 1844, GoB, GD, 1844/34/380, MSA.

[139] From the Asst. Surgeon, Colaba Lunatic Asylum, to the Secretary of the Medical Board, 21 February 1847, GoB, GD, 1847/41, MSA.

[140] *Ganja* is a variation of hemp. Report of the Indian Hemp Drugs Commission, 1894–1895, Vol. 2, p. 182, NLS.

[141] The word 'quack' was inserted after the word *hakim* in the original interview transcript. The addition was probably made by the superintendent.

[142] Report of the Indian Hemp Drugs Commission, 1894–1895, Vol. 2, p. 185, NLS.

[143] Report of the Indian Hemp Drugs Commission, 1894–1895, Vol. 2, p. 186, NLS.

[144] *Bhang, ganja, and charas* are different variations of hemp.

and his brothers and employers knew all about it. The family probably lied about his hemp use because they were afraid of the consequences it would have on Metho.[145] The fact that the family lied showed that they distrusted asylum agencies and wanted to protect their relatives.

The common image of the asylum as a place of confinement for unmanageable mentally ill people obstructed its acceptance as a legitimate medical institution. Dr. Shaw, Superintendent of the Central Lunatic Asylum at Yerawada, deprecated the misconception that the local communities had of the asylum as a place of confinement for the incurable:

> Cases of mental disease are kept at home and treated with quack medicines and charms, mainly because the relatives do not realise that an 'Asylum' is also a 'Hospital'. They are sent to the asylum as a rule incurable, after some years only when the family have given up hope of recovery, and because the patients had become too unmanageable in his home.[146]

In rare cases when families resorted to committing relatives to an asylum, it was meant to be only a temporary relief for them. They did not perceive the asylum as a curative institution. Many families appealed for the discharge or transfer of their relatives, stating that their condition was getting worse in the asylum.[147] While Dr. Shaw hoped that the Indian perception of the asylum would change and the asylum would gain in legitimacy, the growing nationalist movement restrained colonial medical ambitions.[148]

'The emerging processes of nationalist reconstruction of the past and the quest for a new identity as medico-cultural identity' thwarted the efforts of superintendents for improvements and assimilation of the colonial asylum.[149] Dr. Shaw emphasized that 'the chief obstruction to progress in psychiatry in India', despite the poor condition of lunatic asylums, was the 'lack of a definitely expressed public opinion', which delayed improvements. Furthermore, he noted that the Indian masses led by

---

[145] Report of the Indian Hemp Drugs Commission, 1894–1895, Vol. 2, p. 188, NLS.

[146] From the Superintendent, Central Lunatic Asylum, Yerawada, to Surgeon General with the Government of Bombay, 16 July 1920, GoB, GD, 1922/2257B, MSA.

[147] From Bausilal Ramchandra to the Under Secretary to the GoB, Poona, 22 February 1897, GD, 1897/68, MSA.

[148] Poonam Bala, '"Nationalizing" Medicine: The Changing Paradigm of Ayurveda in British India', in Poonam Bala (ed.), *Contesting Colonial Authority: Medicine and Indigenous Responses in Nineteenth and Twentieth-Century India* (Lanham, Boulder, New York, Toronto, Plymouth: Lexington Books, 2012), p. 11.

[149] Bala, '"Nationalizing" Medicine', p. 11.

M.K. Gandhi preferred 'the Ayurvedic and other indigenous systems' for treating mental illness.[150] The emerging nationalist movement, rooted in the conviction of reviving traditional medical systems, frustrated colonial medical hegemonic designs of the superintendents.

CONCLUSION

In the Bombay Presidency, the public perceptions of the asylum hindered its extensive use. The colonial asylum failed to project itself as a curative institution. While medical agencies did their best to protect the image of the asylum and project it as a 'hospital', Indians perceived the asylum as a place for confinement. Bombay's local elite, through philanthropy, collaborated with the government to expand its public health services. The asylum for the local elite was a political and philanthropic avenue. It became a site for projecting their high standing with the colonial state or within their own communities. These elite, however, advocated the asylum's use only for the poor and destitute. The asylum commanded the attention of the press only when it was at the centre of a public scandal. The local press exposed the deplorable conditions of the asylums and influenced public attitudes towards their use. The masses perceived the asylum as a forced intervention in their family life. The links between the asylum and the penal and judicial departments only added to the stigma attached to mental illness. As a result, Indian families took recourse to the asylum only when all other methods of treatment had failed and the person was irrepressible.

On one hand, the *pagal khana* in public opinion was a receptacle for mentally ill people who were unmanageable or dangerous to the larger community. On the other hand, the government refused to make adequate provisions for the patients that Indian communities admitted to the asylum as a last resort. As a result, the condition of the asylums and the public perceptions about them hardly changed. In 1918, the Surgeon General with the Government of Bombay concurred with the local public opinion that the asylum in colonial Bombay was 'little more than its name indicate[d], refuges for insanes'.[151] The lunatic asylum had rightly earned its local name: *pagal khana*.

---

[150] Shaw, 'The Alienist Department of India', p. 334.
[151] From the Surgeon General with the Government of Bombay, No. c. 2173, 21 November 1918, GoB, GD, 1919/1175, MSA.

CHAPTER 7

Conclusion: Shackled Bodies, Unchained Minds

The lunatic asylum was a peripheral yet controversial colonial medical institution. The Superintending Surgeon of Dharwar had rightly postulated that an unregulated asylum system could have negative implications for Indian society (Chap. 6). The trajectory of the Victorian asylum system had influenced his views. Despite government regulations, Victorian asylums had turned into institutions of abuse. His concern that the colonial lunatic asylum might become 'instead of a blessing … a curse to the country', was well founded. This study, by evaluating the implications the lunatic asylum had for the local Indian population, asks if the colonial asylum system had indeed turned into a 'curse' instead of a 'blessing' for the local community.

Historians have used the colonial lunatic asylum archive to analyse colonial motivations[1] in establishing such institutions. This study, instead, has focused on the experience of the Indians with colonial lunatic asylums, bearing in mind James Morris' view. At the zenith of the Raj, he explained, the belief that 'they were performing a divine purpose, innocently nobly,

[1] James Mills argued that the asylum served the Raj for the purposes of the civilizing mission. See James Mills, '"More Important to Civilise than Subdue"? Lunatic Asylums, Psychiatric Practice and Fantasies of the "Civilising Mission" in British India 1858–1900', in Harald Fischer-Tiné and Michael Mann (eds.), *Colonialism as Civilising Mission* (London: Anthem Press, 2003).

© The Author(s) 2018   183
S. A. Pinto, *Lunatic Asylums in Colonial Bombay*,
Mental Health in Historical Perspective,
https://doi.org/10.1007/978-3-319-94244-5_7

184 S. A. PINTO

in the name of God and the Queen' guided colonial motivations.[2] Moreover, colonial agencies had heterogeneous views on the need and purpose of lunatic asylums (Chaps. 2 and 6). By focusing on the Indian experience, the study concludes that irrespective of these varying motivations behind its establishment, the lunatic asylum system, at least in Bombay Presidency, failed to assimilate into Indian society and therefore remained a failed colonial medical enterprise. The book, then, probes the local and colonial factors that contributed to this failure.

In researching the causes of the failure of the asylum system, this historical narrative has accounted for incidences that apparently seem trifling. Historians often neglect such 'trifling', 'common', or 'everyday' incidents because they are 'obvious and immanent'.[3] For example, 'noise' within the asylum is an 'obvious and immanent' fact. However, a closer examination of the aural environment of the asylum proves that it was an unregulated and unregimented domain (Chap. 6). Other examples of 'trifling' evidence are the petitions for the release of family members, which seem to have little significance prima facie. Such petitions, Mills argued, suggested that families were taking back their relatives because they still had productive capacity.[4] Disagreeing with such a proposition, this study argued that these petitions constitute evidence of the lack of trust that Indian families had in the asylum as a curative institution.

In constructing its arguments, this historical narrative has built upon the scholarship of other historians of colonial psychiatry; however, it also fills in gaps in present scholarship. It is the first comprehensive history of lunatic asylums in the Bombay Presidency from 1793 to 1921. In terms of regional history writing, extant scholarship has largely dealt with the history of asylums in North India. In these asylums, although superintendents adopted hybrid treatment practices, historians have argued that by 1912 these became 'colonial archetypes'.[5] However, the asylums in the Bombay Presidency, as this book argues, remained 'imperfectly designed

---

[2] Ashish Nandy, *The Intimate Enemy: Loss and Recovery of Self Under Colonialism* (Delhi: Oxford University Press, 1983), p. 34.

[3] Gyanendra Pandey, 'Unarchived Histories: The "Mad" and the "Trifling"', in Gyanendra Pandey (ed.), *Unarchived Histories: The "Mad" and the "Trifling" in the Colonial and Postcolonial World* (London and New York: Routledge, 2014), pp. 7–8.

[4] James Mills, *Madness, Cannabis and Colonialism: The 'Native-Only' Lunatic Asylums of British India, 1857–1900* (Basingstoke: Macmillan Press Limited, 2000), p. 140.

[5] Anouska Bhattacharyya, 'Indian Insanes, Lunacy in the "Native" Asylums of Colonial India, 1858–1912', PhD Thesis, Harvard University, 2013, p. 206.

institutions'—'poorly equipped' and 'imperfectly staffed'.[6] Moreover, scholars have also argued that starting from the mid-nineteenth century, Indian lunatic asylums experienced a 'huge transformation' and after 1912, 'behaved in a coordinated and homogenous' manner.[7] Bombay's lunatic asylums clearly swerved from this model, lagging both in profit making and in the adoption of 'modern' methods of treatment. As a colonial medical institution, Bombay's lunatic asylums were negotiated spaces rather than 'colonial archetypes'.[8]

BOMBAY'S LUNATIC ASYLUMS: 'A NEGOTIATED SPACE'

An examination of the nature of the colonial asylum system reveals the complexities of colonial medical encounters. The book expounded on these complexities by arguing that the asylums represented a 'middle ground'. The third chapter highlighted the state of a fragmented colonial bureaucracy that differed in their understandings of the functions of the asylum. These divisions paved the way for negotiations with Indian staff, families and patients.

The asylum became a middle ground in the colony as superintendents, staff, patients, and local communities negotiated with each other to meet 'specific ends'.[9] Patients, however, had the least negotiating power. European superintendents permitted these negotiations because it was necessary for the survival of the asylum system. Keeping in line with Roy Porter, this book highlights the character of the lunatic asylum as a 'contested site' of 'constant negotiations'.[10] These negotiations ensured that the asylum evaded colonial hegemony; the asylum even in the twentieth century did not change into a 'colonial bastion',[11] as Indians never accepted its legitimacy or efficacy. However, the negotiations took place

[6] From the Surgeon General with the Government of Bombay, 21 November 1918, GoB, GD, 1919/ 1175, MSA.

[7] Bhattacharyya, 'Indian Insanes, Lunacy in the "Native" Asylums of Colonial India', p. 206.

[8] Ibid., p. 206.

[9] Richard White, *The Middle Ground: Indians, Empires, and Republics in the Great Lakes Region, 1650–1815* (Cambridge: Cambridge University Press, 1991), p. 51.

[10] Roy Porter, 'Introduction', in Roy Porter and David Wright (eds.), *The Confinement of the Insane: International Perspectives, 1800–1965* (New York: Cambridge University Press, 2003), p. 5.

[11] Bhattacharyya, 'Indian Insanes, Lunacy in the "Native" Asylums of Colonial India', p. 206.

within a context of an uneven relationship of power. Therefore, although asylum agencies failed to achieve hegemony, they nonetheless exerted various forms of control over the patients.

The book in this context has re-evaluated the agency of superintendents. Superintendents were not passive colonial agents. The third chapter highlighted the ambiguity in the relationship between the European superintendent and the colonial state. Different colonial agencies had varying perceptions of the functions of lunatic asylums, and superintendents did not always subscribe to the government's vision. Some superintendents did show a humanitarian concern in their interaction with the Indian staff and patients. They displayed a sense of empathy towards them, supporting petitions for better facilities for their staff and yielding at times to patient's requests. Superintendents even negotiated treatment practices within the asylum.

Superintendents conceded to administering treatment to patients on the 'common-sense' principle (Chap. 4). The common-sense treatment of Indian insanity was a hybrid method of treating patients with clothing, food, and occupation. Local conditions and financial expediency affected the ways in which superintendents implemented such methods. Examples of negotiations in treatment practices included permitting a money allowance for patients who refused to eat, or appointing a Brahmin cook, or the use of Indian attire as uniforms for patients. By the twentieth century, superintendents argued that the 'common-sense' method was best suited for Indian patients. These superintendents even resisted the implementation of western medicine and treatment practices in Bombay's asylums (Chap. 4). The failure of the hegemonic designs of western medicine and the development of the asylum as a negotiated space are also evident in its soundscape.

Asylum staff failed to achieve sonic hegemony in Bombay's asylums, as local Indian languages dominated the soundscape (Chap. 5). Moreover, these asylums featured unregulated and unregimented soundscapes. Financial expediency restrained the efforts of superintendents in silencing patients. They relied instead on physically exhausting patients through labour to quieten them. Superintendents failed in achieving hegemony over the asylums' aural environment. Their willingness to negotiate with families also defeated colonial hegemonic designs.

In order to accommodate the wishes of families, superintendents often compromised on the regular medical code. One example would be Dr. Campbell's discharge of patients before they were 'perfectly convalescent'.

Superintendents felt that such negotiations were necessary in order to influence the perception of the local community about the asylum. However, despite the efforts of superintendents, the local community perceived the asylum as a place of permanent confinement (Chap. 6). Several forms of negotiations were evident in the everyday running of the asylum. These negotiations, however, had their limitations, and therefore barely alleviated the historical trauma experienced by the patients or their families.

HISTORICAL TRAUMA, INDIAN SOCIETY, AND THE LUNATIC ASYLUM

The main aim of this study is to account for the historical traumas associated with lunatic asylums in the Bombay Presidency. These traumas occurred even though the asylum was a negotiated site or 'middle ground'.[12] Moreover, such historical trauma explains the aversion of the Indians towards colonial asylums and to mental hospitals even today, since these traumas are intergenerational.[13] As noted earlier, the book does not examine the colonial motivations for establishing the asylum; it has instead explored the lived experiences of patients and local communities as they encountered a foreign medical institution. Irrespective of colonial motivations, these institutions caused 'soul wounds' to local communities. Although for a few local groups like asylum staff or the elite the institution was a means of personal gain, the general masses resisted the assimilation of the colonial lunatic asylum because of the 'soul wounds' they experienced. This study explains these wounds through six related themes.

The first of these themes is the undermining of Indian worldviews, medical practitioners, and caretakers by colonial agencies. In examining the causes of the failure of the asylum system, the book began by analysing the ideological setting within which the colonial lunatic asylum was established. The interwoven spiritual-somatic Indian perspectives on mental illness and its treatment contested this ideological foundation of the asylum system (Chap. 2). The Victorian asylum as a mental institution was a result of a separation of the spiritual and somatic meanings of mental

---

[12] Richard White, *The Middle Ground: Indians, Empires, and Republics in the Great Lakes Region, 1650–1815* (Cambridge: Cambridge University Press, 1991).

[13] Eduardo Duran, *Healing the Soul Wound: Counselling with American Indian and Other Native People* (New York: Teachers College Press, 2006), p. 16.

illness. This separation gave psychiatrists their legitimacy as professionals.[14] Indian ideas of insanity and its treatment starkly contrasted with the colonial approach to mental illness. To propagate the use of the asylum, colonial agencies projected Indian treatment practices as stagnant and superstitious. Such a colonial narrative served to normalize the colonial position, based on the supposed superiority of western medicine. However, it failed to convince the local communities to seek treatment at an asylum. Indian society came to consider the asylum system and European doctors as interfering in their socio-religious customs and practices. The process of establishing and maintaining the asylum system also undermined the position of the practitioners of Indian medicine. Indian doctors were labelled quacks, and religious mendicants like *sadhus* and *fakirs*, associated with the care of people who suffered from mental illness, were themselves incarcerated.

The second theme studied is the colonial interference in close family and community ties. The lunatic asylum as a by-product of individualistic societies in England was irrelevant to Indian society that valued its close family ties (Chap. 2). The asylum system failed to assimilate into Indian society because it rejected Indian notions of insanity and its collective approach to caring for mentally ill people. In Indian society, mentally ill people were cared for within their families and communities. The asylum system forced their separation from them. In collectivistic societies, there are intrinsic links between the individual and the group or community; this separation caused trauma to both the families involved and the patients. For Indian families, then, the asylum represented a forced and undesirable intervention into their traditional family and community lives.

The third theme examined is the undermining of Indian culture. Scholars have drawn considerable attention to the role of the asylum in exerting control over the Indian body.[15] This study has also argued that the asylum was a space for the execution of a 'cultural project of control'[16] (Chap. 4). Asylum agencies forced patients to conform to colonial perceptions of an Indian subject. For example, the use of uniform asylum attire

---

[14] Andrew Scull, *Madness in Civilization: A Cultural History of Insanity, from the Bible to Freud, from the Madhouse to Modern Medicine* (Princeton and Oxford: Princeton University Press, 2015); Andrew Scull, 'From Madness to Mental Illness: Medical Men as Moral Entrepreneurs', *European Journal of Sociology*, Vol. 16, No. 2, 1975, p. 254.

[15] Mills, *Madness, Cannabis and Colonialism*, p. 110.

[16] Nicholas Dirks, 'Foreword', in Bernard Cohn, *Colonialism and its Forms of Knowledge: The British in India* (New Jersey: Princeton University Press, 1996), p. ix.

was culturally insensitive, considering the fact that for local people their heterogeneous attire was a symbol of their identity.[17] Colonial agencies often misunderstood Indian cultural practices; for example, the Hindu practice of ritual fasting became a cause for incarcerating Brahmin Devram (Chap. 3). Ex-patient Sajan Curim could have been right to some extent when he complained that 'only twenty per cent of the patients are actually insane'.[18] Miss Sheppard, the Chaplain of the Colaba Lunatic Asylum, echoed the same view.[19]

The fourth theme discussed in this book is that the colonial asylum was a source of trauma for patients who were physically and mentally weak but had to labour. Indian insanity was treated in a 'common-sense' way; this included clothing, feeding, and occupying patients (Chap. 4). Superintendents adopted this method as a practical means to manage Indian insanity and such treatment methods helped in alleviating the monetary burden of the state. However, the government reduced budgets at the cost of patient welfare. As Superintendent Niven explained, the asylum provided patients with 'too much treatment and too little care'.[20] Superintendents faced constant pressure not only to maintain the 'asylum efficiency logic',[21] but also to maximize profits. The government and asylum agencies often prioritized profits over the care of patients. Clothing and diet treatment served to prepare the Indian body for labour rather than cure patients. At times asylum staff refused to provide medicine due to shortage of funds, and at other times to keep patients alert for work. On the pretext of treating them, superintendents lent patients out to the PWD and other government institutions to offer labour. Such asylum 'treatment' practices were a cause for families keeping their relatives who suffered from mental illness homebound rather than admitting them to an asylum.

[17] Emma Tarlo, *Clothing Matters: Dress and Identity in India* (Chicago: University of Chicago Press, 1996), p. 13.

[18] From Sajan Curim to the Secretary to the Government of Bombay, 16 October 1893, GoB, GD, 1893/75, MSA.

[19] From Miss Mary Shepherd to the Governor in Council, 31 May 1904, GoB, GD, 1904/57, MSA.

[20] Dr. Niven, Superintendent of the Colaba Lunatic Asylum, noted that while the Lunacy Acts made provisions for the 'care and treatment' of patients in lunatic asylums, most often, 'poor lunatics' received 'too much treatment and too little care'. APR, 1873–1874, p. 21, NLS, Scotland.

[21] Roman et al., 'No Time for Nostalgia!: Asylum-making, Medicalized Colonialism in British Columbia (1859–97) and Artistic Praxis for Social Transformation', *International Journal of Qualitative Studies in Education*, Vol. 22, No. 1, 2009, p. 34.

A fifth trauma identified in this book is the manipulation of patients' voices. Asylum agencies, manipulated patients' voices, adding to their trauma both behind and beyond asylum walls (Chap. 5). The impairment of a group's ability 'to speak and be heard'[22] was a form of epistemic violence that clearly manifested itself in the asylum. Asylum staff and other colonial agencies used patients' voices for their medical and evidential value. They manipulated the patients' ability 'to speak and be heard' in two ways. First, they physically obstructed patients, preventing them from making complaints to the Visitors. Second, they used their voices as evidence of their mental illness. In the case of an ex-patient, Sajan Curim, who had managed to write a letter of complaint to government authorities, the superintendent used his letter as evidence of his mental illness. Patient silences were also selectively interpreted (Chaps. 4 and 5), sometimes as a symptom of mental illness and on occasions as a sign of improvement. The asylum violated the rights of its patients by controlling the extent to which they could speak and be heard.

The sixth theme discussed is the issue of stigma associated with the asylum, which scholars have largely neglected. Bhattacharyya argued that there was 'no evidence of stigma' associated with the asylum.[23] However, this study, disagreeing with such a proposition, argues that there was a social stigma attached to the use of the asylum (Chap. 6). Moreover, as the government linked asylum committal to the criminal justice system, it further stigmatized asylum use. Bombay's superintendents, in their asylum reports and letters, complained of families refusing to use the asylum because of the stigma associated with it. The constant appeals of families to withdraw relatives from the asylum provide further evidence of stigma attached to the asylum. Public certification of those deemed mentally ill aggravated the shame associated with the asylum's use. The asylum also instilled a sense of fear. Families feared forceful incarceration and permanent confinement of their relatives (Chap. 6). The tendency of families to conceal mental illness was an indication that they feared police incarceration of kin, behind asylum walls.

Finally, considering these Indian experiences of historical trauma or 'soul wounds' associated with the asylum, the book argues that the 'apa-

---

[22] Kirstie Dotson, 'Tracking Epistemic Violence, Tracking Practices of Silences', *Hypatia*, Vol. 26, No. 2, 2011, p. 236.

[23] Bhattacharyya, 'Indian Insanes, Lunacy in the "Native" Asylums of Colonial India', p. 31.

thy' or aversion of Indian society towards lunatic asylums can be understood as resistance. This resistance can be categorized as 'everyday resistances' which 'avoids direct symbolic confrontation with authority or with elite norms'; its weapons, as James Scott argued, are 'foot dragging, dissimulation, false compliance, pilfering, feigned ignorance, slander'.[24] The aversion of the local communities represented a form of 'individual self-help' used by 'powerless groups' (the local community). The lunatic asylum in Bombay was not 'quickly accepted',[25] as communities resisted its legitimization by avoiding its use.

This book accounts for local experiences of the lunatic asylum from 1793 to 1921. Using the colonial lunatic asylum archive, it deliberates on the socio-cultural, spiritual, psychological, and physical impact that the lunatic asylum had on indigenous life. The lunatic asylum was a negotiated space and few benefitted from its establishment; but for those deemed mentally ill and for the masses, it was a place of 'insulation, mystery and darkness'. The 'imperfectly designed'[26] lunatic asylum led to the 'psychological uprooting' and 'cultural disruptions' of Indian communities.[27]

MENTAL HOSPITALS IN MAHARASHTRA TODAY

The Report of the United Nations Special Rapporteur, 28 March 2017, called for a revolution in mental health care. The mental health care system, explained Dr. Dainius Pūras, was in a 'crisis'. He identified problems of power asymmetries, overreliance on psychotropic drugs, and a system that revolves around 'profits' of the experts and pharma industry. These issues have culminated into a coercive and largely biomedical approach to mental health care. Such coercion in the mental health care system, as this study shows, is historically endemic. In the Report, Dr. Pūras calls for

---

[24] James Scott, *Weapons of the Weak: Everyday Forms of Peasant Resistance* (New Haven: Yale University Press, 1985), p. 29, in Douglas Haynes and Gyan Prakash (eds.), *Resistance and Everyday Social Relations in South Asia* (Delhi: Oxford University Press, 1991), pp. 9–10.
[25] Bhattacharyya, 'Indian Insanes, Lunacy in the 'Native' Asylums of Colonial India', p. 31.
[26] From the Surgeon General with the Government of Bombay, 21 November 1918, GoB, GD, 1919/1175, MSA.
[27] Nandy, *The Intimate Enemy*, p. 31.

'bold action' from 'within the corridors of power' and an urgent shift to a 'rights-based' approach to mental health care.[28]

This book, by acknowledging the historical traumas experienced by patients and the local community, intends to create awareness among mental health practitioners and policy makers so that they can initiate 'rights-based' changes in the mental health system. This study aims to disrupt the legacy of historical trauma: patterns of coercion and power asymmetries. It simultaneously paves the way for new narratives in mental health treatment. It intends to help mental health practitioners, policy makers, and Indian society invent better ways to help people suffering from mental illness.

Such a rethinking is necessary, as mental hospitals in Maharashtra today still act as carriers of colonial asylum cultures. Hospital staff unconsciously participate in the continued infliction of 'soul wounds' on patients. Even treatment practices primarily revolve around clothing, feeding, and occupying patients. The Ratnagiri Mental Hospital, the oldest surviving of the three hospitals (under the colonial Bombay Presidency), provides evidence of these forms of treatment. In this hospital, the staff continue to use some of the colonial asylum practices. The hospital does not have a psychiatrist. The Hospital Report for 2013 mentioned clothing, feeding, and occupying patients as its main forms of treatment. The list of activities for patients includes '*bagh wuh sheti kaam*' (gardening and agricultural work), candle-making, stationery file making, screen printing, making other small goods like Diwali lamps, lanterns, and such. Amusement is also part of treatment; however, it involves treating patients like children. Patient activities that consist of indoor and outdoor games reflect the colonial attitude. Games include lime-and-spoon balancing game, pinning the tail on the donkey, running, jumping, and eating *jalebi* (an Indian confectionary). The hospital staff, in implementing such treatment practices, participate actively, yet unconsciously, in perpetuating a colonial practice.

At the Yerawada Mental Hospital, the abuse of patients who refuse to work is evidence of a continuing culture of coercion within hospitals.[29] In

---

[28] Report of the Special Rapporteur on the Right of Everyone to the Enjoyment if the Highest Attainable Standard of Physical and Mental health, Human Rights Council, 28 March 2017, Thirty-Fifth Session, 6–23 June 2017, pp. 5–6; 'World needs "revolution" in mental health care', 6 June 2017, http://www.ohchr.org/en/NewsEvents/Pages/DisplayNews.aspx?NewsID=21689&LangID=E; accessed 15 August 2017.

[29] *The Indian Express*, 23 December 2014; http://indianexpress.com/article/mumbai/in-urgent-need-of-being-human-mental-hospitals/; accessed 27 October 2016.

colonial asylums, labour of patients was crucial to the maintenance of the institution. Even though there is no financial need for patients to labour or perform domestic chores these days, hospital staff force them to put in physical labour and adhere to the belief that such a practice is a necessity. Erving Goffman's argument rightly describes the condition at Maharashtra's mental hospitals: 'Inmates and lower staff levels are involved in a vast supportive action – an elaborate dramatized tribute – that has the effect, if not purpose, of affirming that a medical like service is in progress here and the psychiatric staff are providing it'. As hospital staff continue to adhere to a clothing, feeding, occupying treatment regime, it solidifies their 'self-conception' of providing curative treatment to patients.[30] While there are several continuities in the character of mental hospitals, a few changes have occurred in its environment.

The aural environment of mental hospitals has undergone a significant change in recent years. The use of drugs has silenced the once noisy asylum soundscape. However, the staff continue to lock up patients, despite the use of drugs. The government has made a few alterations to the old building structures that the British had originally designed for custody rather than cure of the patients. Yet, mental hospitals in Maharashtra today continue to perform a custodial function, in lieu of a curative one. Therefore a new approach to mental health, getting away from the colonial paradigm, is urgently necessary in India.

FINAL NOTES

While this research contributes to the scholarship on colonial lunatic asylums, several associated themes await investigation. There is a need to take a regional, rather than national, approach while examining colonial lunatic asylums, since local factors significantly affected the growth, development, and character of these asylums. Moreover, the experiences of women in the asylum—a largely neglected theme—is in need of further examination. A historiographical gap also exists regarding the impact of lunacy laws on the stigmatization of mental illness in colonial India and the effect of colonialism on Indian mental health.

This book, in accounting for the Indian experience of the lunatic asylum, began by examining their ideological understanding of insanity and

[30] Erving Goffman, *Asylums: Essays on the Social Situation of Mental Patients and Other Inmates* (New York: Anchor Books, 1961), p. 385.

treatment practices. It then moved to an examination of the nature of the lunatic asylum, its treatment practices, and the asylum soundscape. Finally, it analysed Indian perceptions of the asylum. Through an analysis of these colonial and local factors, the book has argued that the colonial lunatic asylum failed to assimilate into Indian society and therefore remained a failed colonial medical enterprise. The words of the Superintending Surgeon of Dharwar regarding the dangers of the asylum system summarize the Indian experience of the lunatic asylum. In the experience of the Indians, except for the staff and the elite who gained from its establishment, the lunatic asylum was indeed 'instead of a blessing … a curse'.[31]

---

[31] From the Superintending Surgeon, Dharwar to the Secretary to the Medical Board, 15 March 1845, GoB, GD, 1845/43-94, MSA.

APPENDIX 1

Source: Author's Photographs, November–December 2014

THANA REGIONAL MENTAL HOSPITAL (FORMERLY KNOWN AS THE NAROTAMDAS MADHAVDAS LUNATIC ASYLUM)

© The Author(s) 2018
S. A. Pinto, *Lunatic Asylums in Colonial Bombay*,
Mental Health in Historical Perspective,
https://doi.org/10.1007/978-3-319-94244-5

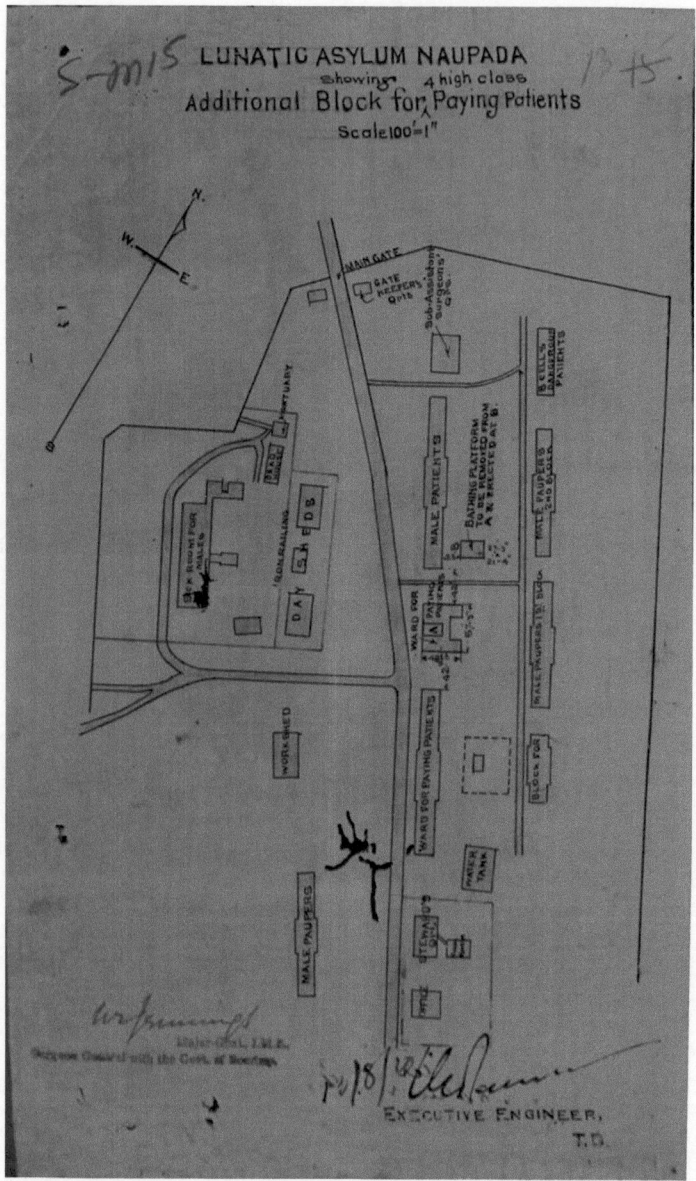

Fig. A.1 Plan of the NMLA, Thana. (Source: From the Superintendent to the Executive Engineer, 14 May 1920, GoB, GD, 1920/1139, MSA)

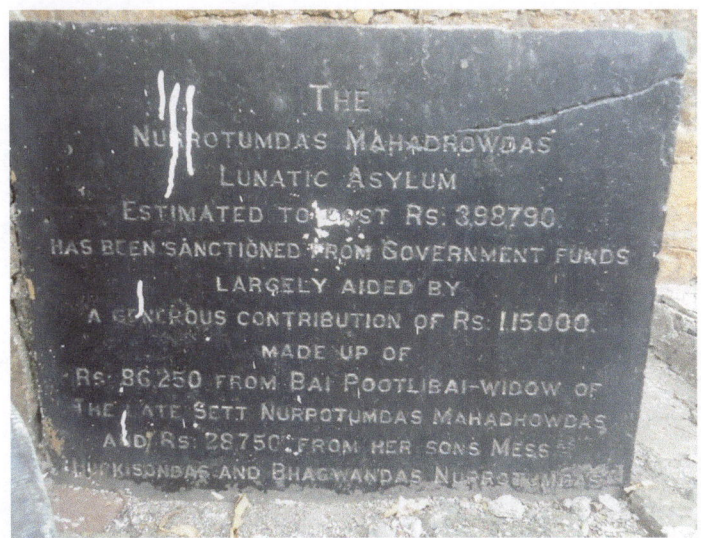

Fig. A.2 Marble stone tablet installed at Thana Regional Mental Hospital (TRH), Mumbai

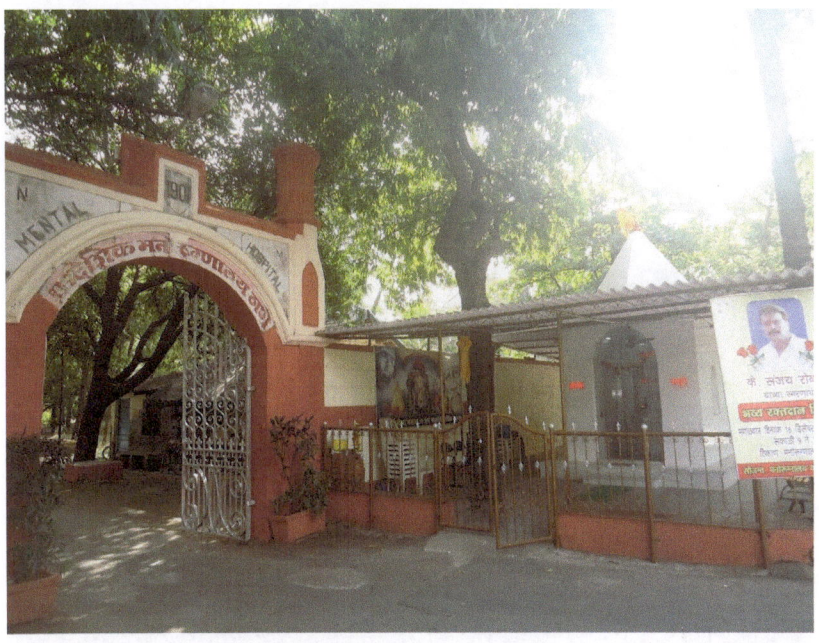

Fig. A.3 Main Gate, TRH

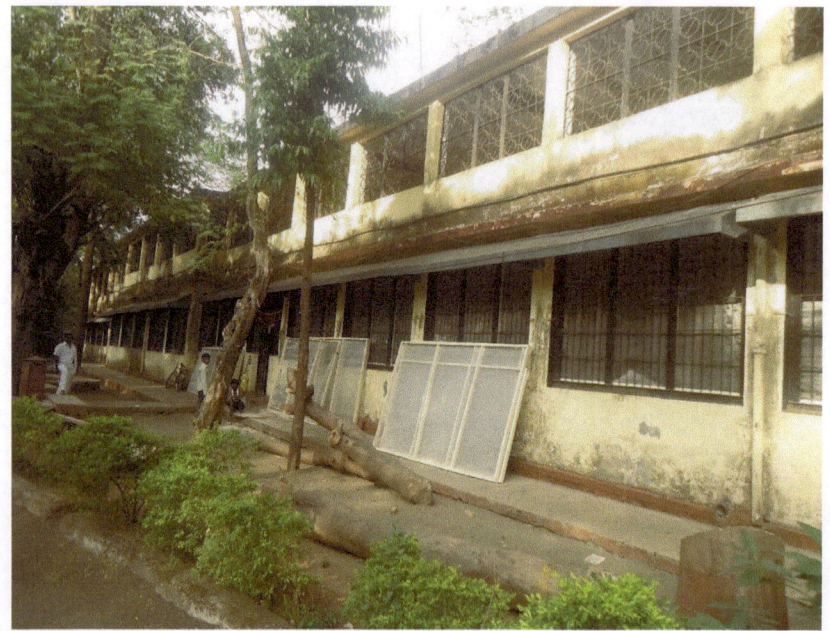

Fig. A.4 Main men's ward, TRH

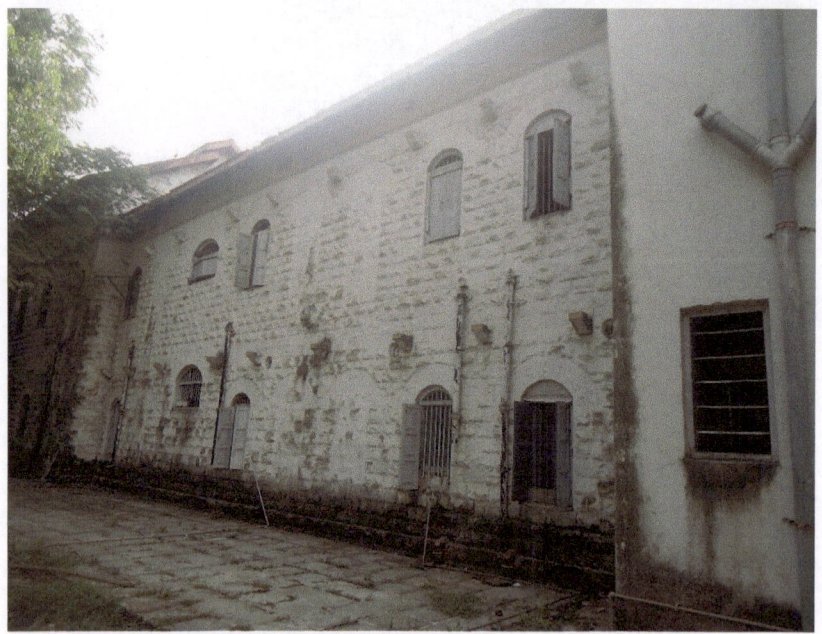

Fig. A.5 Rear view of the main men's ward, TRH

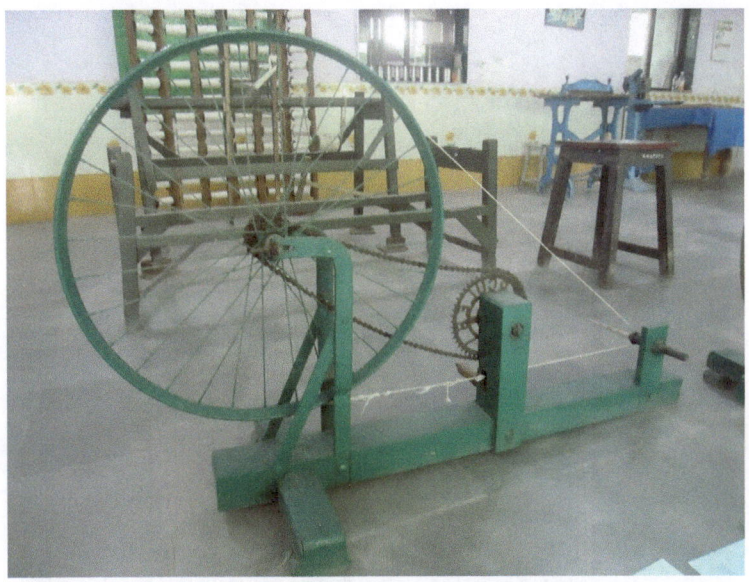

Fig. A.6 *Charkha* or spinning wheel, used for occupational therapy

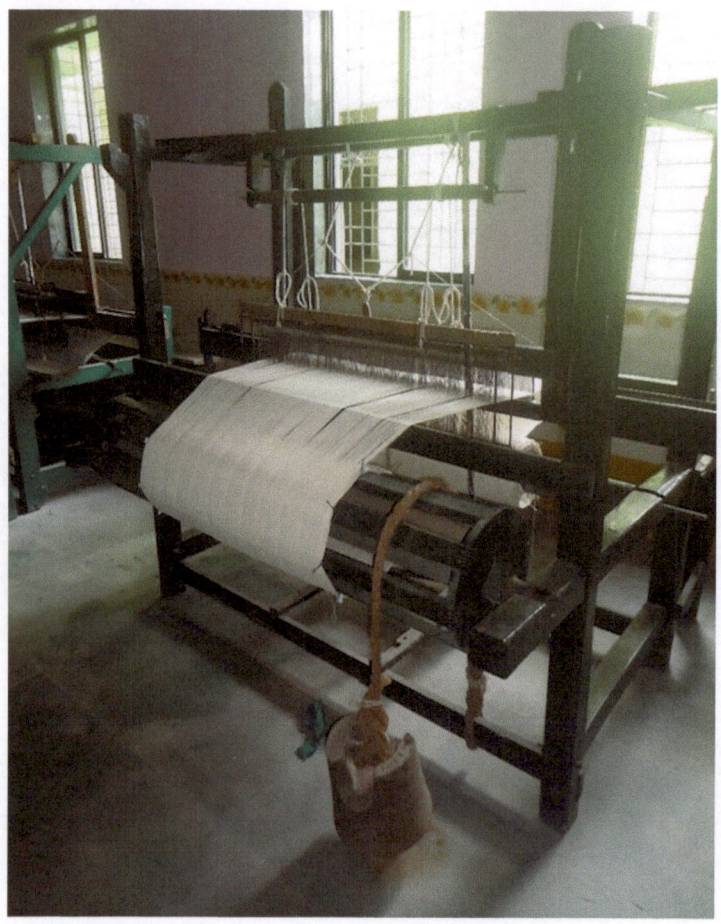

Fig. A.7 Weaving machine used for occupational therapy, installed by asylum authorities when the asylum was first established in 1902

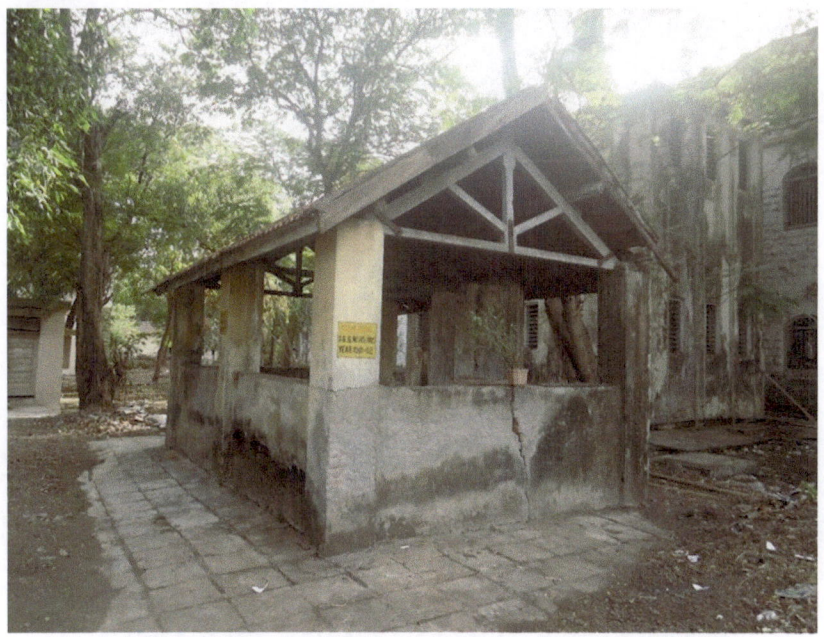

Fig. A.8   The work shed, TRH

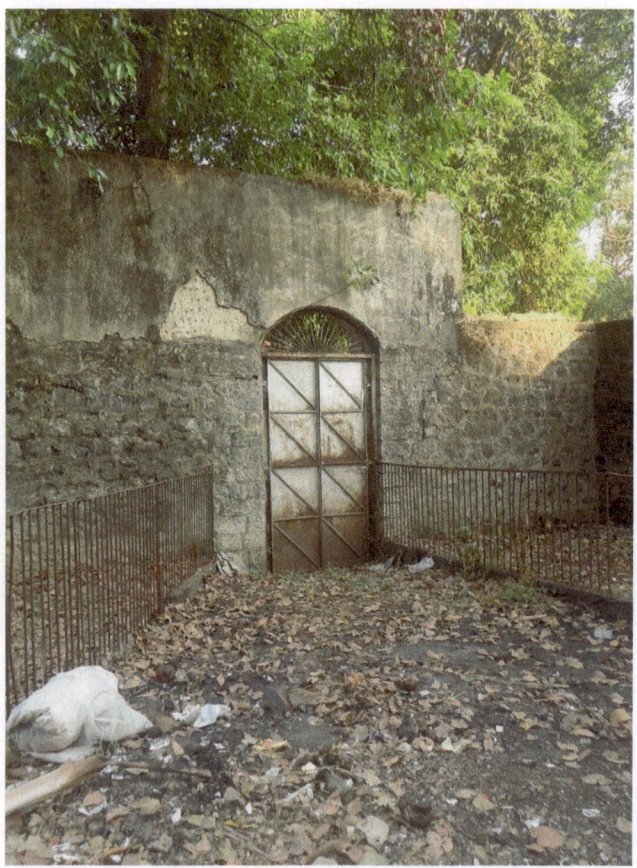

Fig. A.9   The side gate at the TRH, which is used for the dead. The gate is an example of the inclusion of the local custom of not taking a dead body through the main door. The gate also provides architectural evidence for the character of the asylum as a middle ground

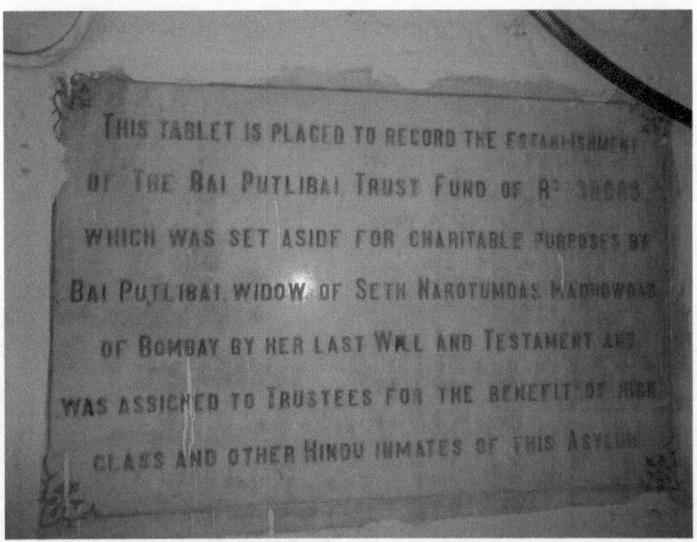

Fig. A.10 Stone tablet outside the Superintendent's office in recognition of the trust fund set up by the Madhavdas family

Ratnagiri Regional Mental Hospital (Formerly Known as the Ratnagiri Lunatic Asylum)

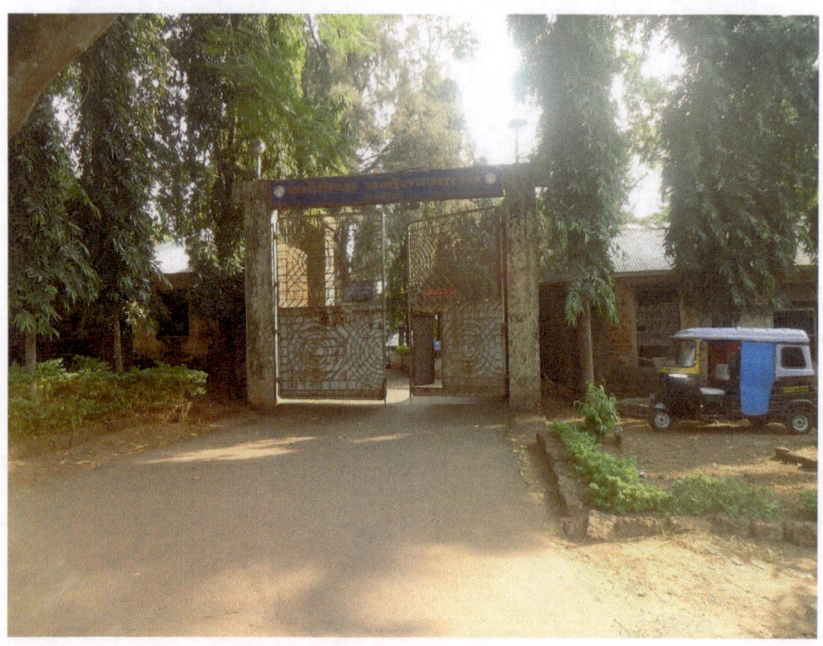

Fig. A.11   Main Gate, Ratnagiri Mental Hospital (RMH)

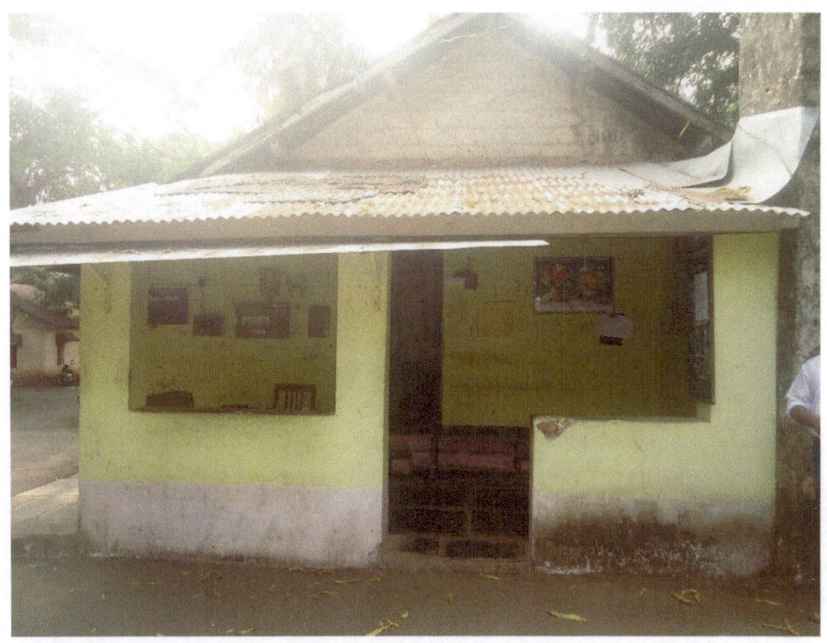

Fig. A.12 The office in which patients are first evaluated on their arrival, RMH

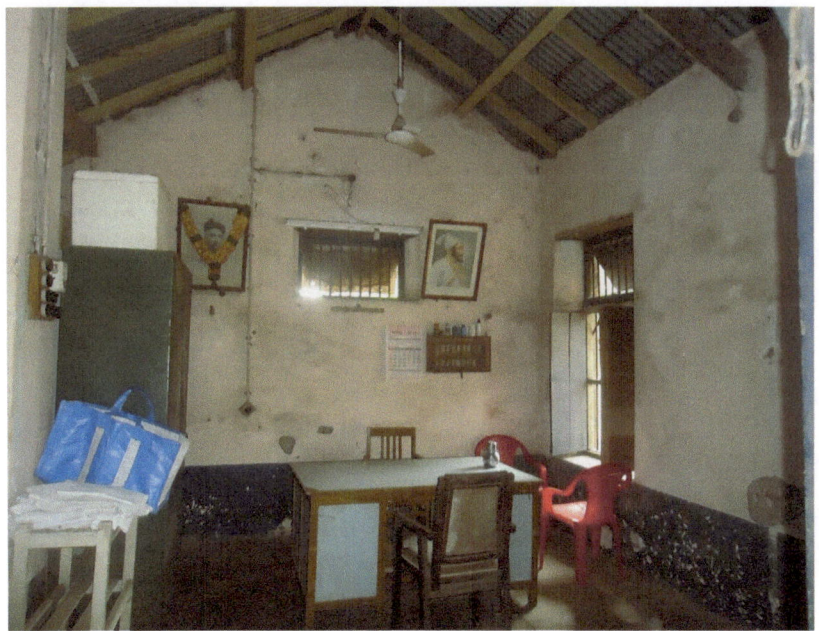

Fig. A.13 Interiors of the same office

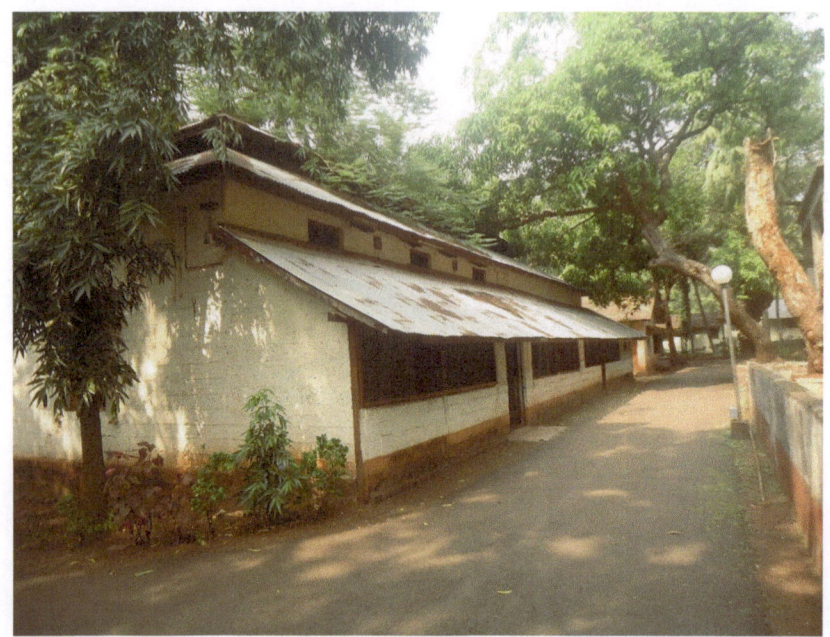

Fig. A.14 The men's ward, RMH

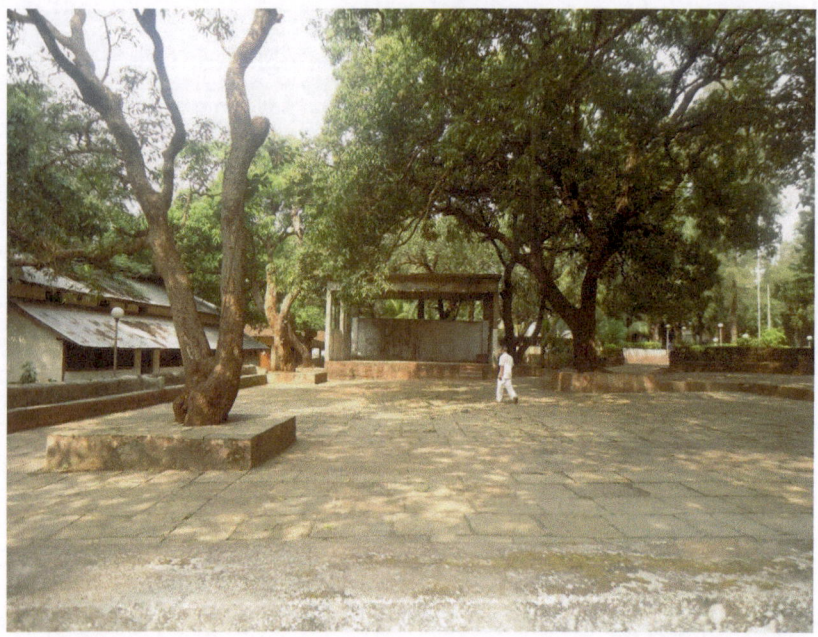

Fig. A.15 The space used for amusement, RMH

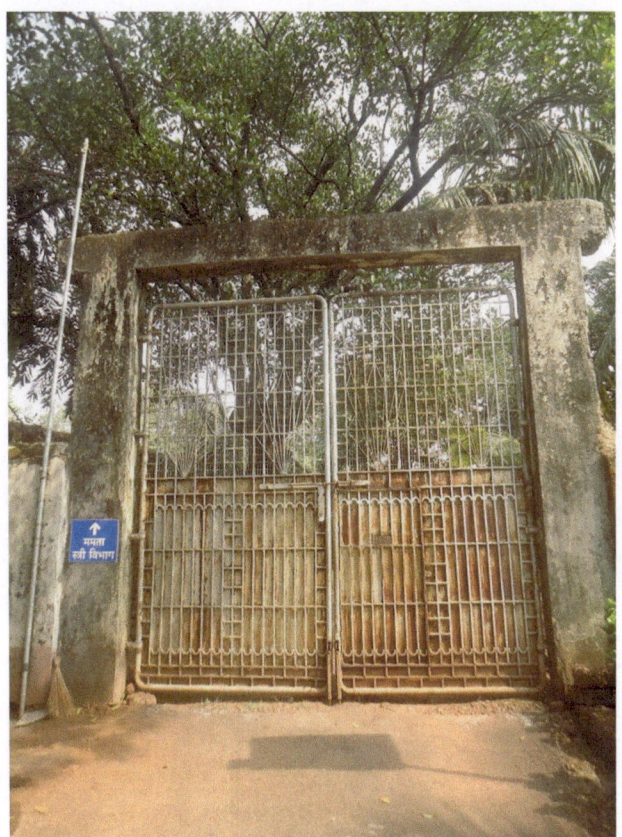

Fig. A.16   The gate to the women's section, RMH

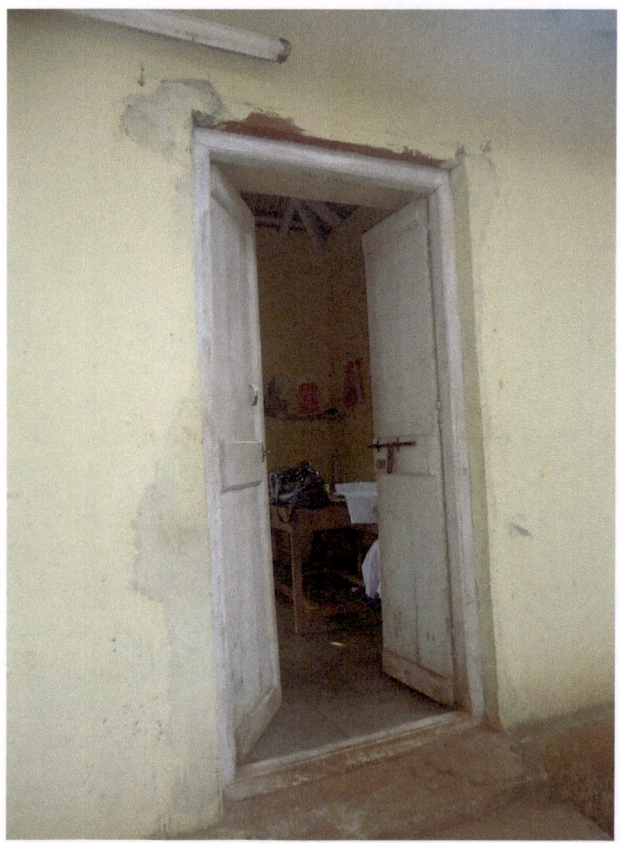

Fig. A.17 Door to a small room that provides access to the women's section, RMH. Food is supplied through this door. It also serves as a pick-up point for food

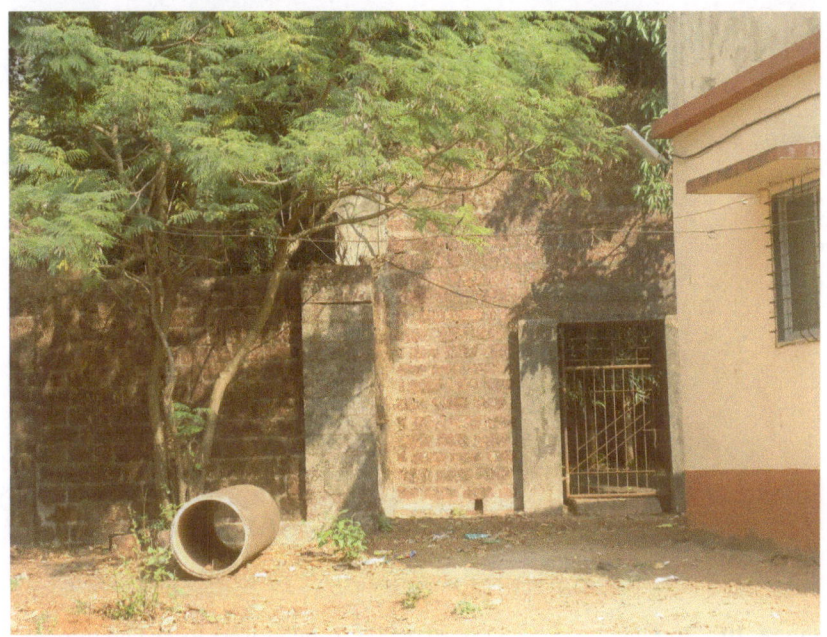

Fig. A.18 The side gate, RMH

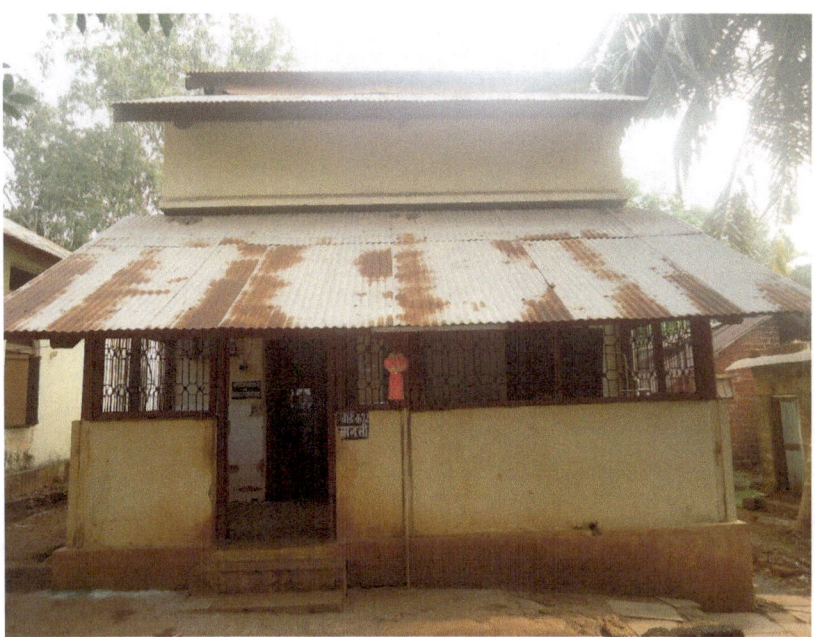

Fig. A.19 Women's infirmary, RMH

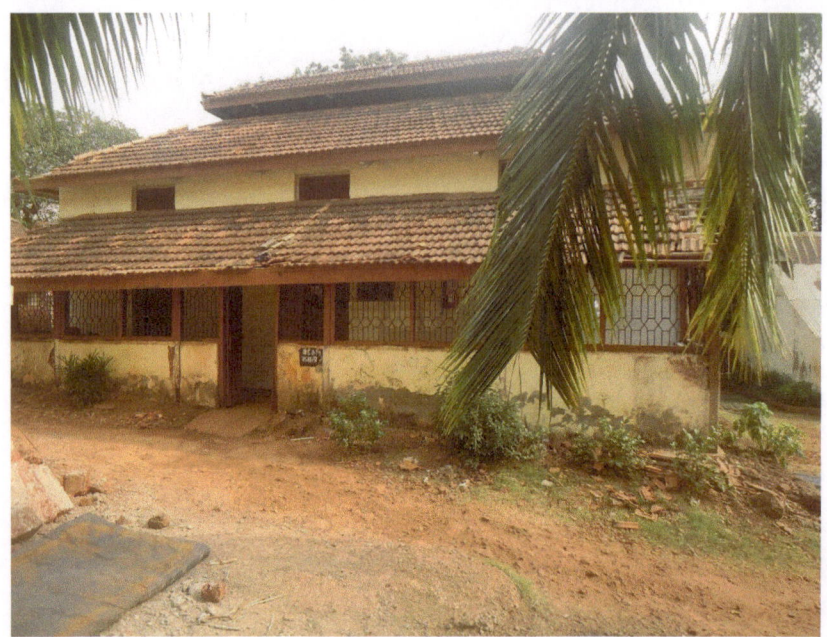

Fig. A.20 *Manali,* the women's ward, RMH. Patients were locked up throughout the day in this ward and were let out only during meal times or for work

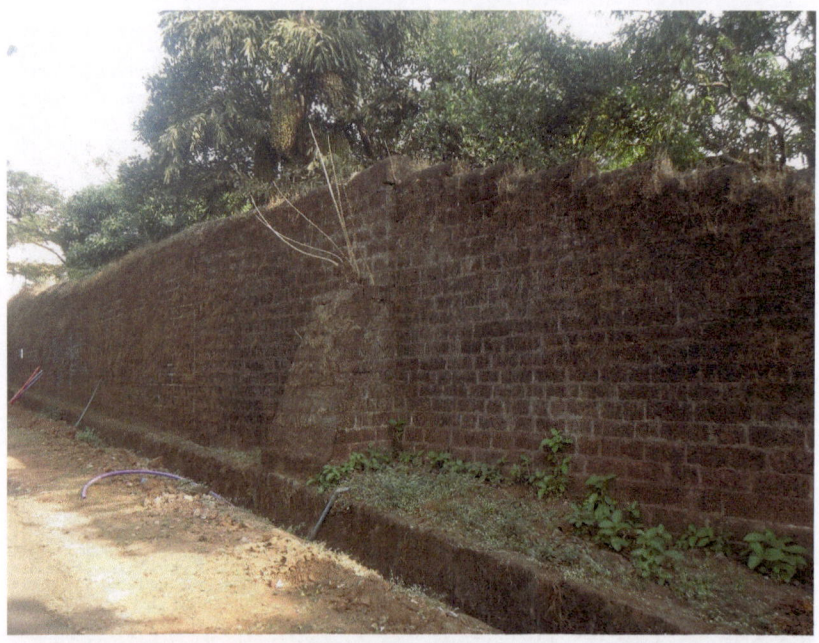

Fig. A.21 The exterior wall around the hospital, built in 1886, proves the custodial intent in constructing the asylum

Appendix 2

Letter from Ex-Patient Sajan Curim to the Superintendent, Colaba Lunatic Asylum, 1891 (sic)

In the month of February 8th morning about 9 o'clock from my self-confinement against my judgement creditors.

Mr. Vergee Damjee asked me to drive out in the hired Victoria with Mr Cursetjess Dadabhoy Khansaheb and Khan Mohamed Sherif Curm of Messrs. Sherff Son and Company.

So we all went up to lower Colaba at soda water shop drunk there syrup with ice soda, payment made by Khan Mohamed Sherif.

Thence from the Doctor's bungalow being in the side of Colaba Lunatic Asylum. After fifteen minitues I saw one chopped hand European with two portugues, the said European sat on chair, and asked me if I pay you money will you sign a receipt for the same? I said after reading the receipt in mean time he put his head on his hand on the table without speaking a word to anyone.

I and co-passengers left the bungalow and drived up to appear near "Sassoon Dock."

On my checking the driver for having driven on vacant Pear Road turned his carriage to the door of the Hospital. I hence entered within the gate, my uncle Mr Veerjee called me out, O replied after seeing the hospital we will go together at home, near the hospital office, a European (Kelly) came out and told me the doctor is coming for you and he put me underlocked and asked for my turban and white coat called ungharakha.

© The Author(s) 2018
S. A. Pinto, *Lunatic Asylums in Colonial Bombay*,
Mental Health in Historical Perspective,
https://doi.org/10.1007/978-3-319-94244-5

At night by their wardboys opened my lock and [gave me a] small cup of fenny. I asked water to dilute, they refused and beat me hard.

On the 9th of February at 8 o'clock in the morning, a European who I saw at the doctors bungalow came before me where I [was] lock[ed] up [on] my asking he said he possess plenty of money, I told him better way to call my books.

This question remained silence up last, and I tried up to 12th June 1890, 8 o'clock in the morning left the hospital with my brother Mr Jan Mohamed Curim.

SAJAN CURIM,

The Ecclesiastical and Mania Chronic[1]

LETTER FROM EX-PATIENT SAJAN CURIM TO THE GOVERNMENT OF BOMBAY, 1893 (SIC)

Sir,

I beg respectfully to bring to the notice of the government the following facts relating to the Colaba Lunatic Asylum which has come under my observation.

I was an inmate of this Asylum twice according to my account. Viz. 8/2 to 30/5/88 + 4/7/88 to 12/6/90

During the time of Dr. Niven, the management of the Asylum was proper. He used to come himself in company with the relatives of the inmates, ask questions, see wether the malady had increased or decreased,+ he satisfied himself that everything pertaining to their comfort was right in every case.

I am reported to have been "Ecclesiastical and Mania Chronic". What this means [I do not know]

The act relating to the establishment of Asylums defines a "lunatic" a person of "unsound mind, or idiot." But in my case, I have been examined by medical practitioners prior to my admission into the Asylum, and pronounced me as perfectly sane, Their names are Dr Anna Moreshwar Kunte, M.D, Dr. A.G.Viegas.

It is only wandering and dangerous lunatics who are taken into custody and sent by a magistrate to the Asylum. After a medical officer examines him and signs a medical certificate.

I wrote to the superintendent of the Asylum to let me have a copy of the certificate of my admission, signed by a medical officer but as yet, I have not

---

[1] From Sajan Curim to the Superintendent, Colaba Lunatic Asylum, 17 October 1891, GoB, GD, 1893/75, MSA.

been furnished witte one, strange to say. My own opinion is that really speaking, twenty percent inmates are only insane, the rest cannot with propriety be called as such, as they are driven to this abode by some freak of fortune. And the visitors of the asylum hardly inquire into this matter, As when they attend the stewards, apothecary surgeon, are in front and they do not allow any complaint to go to them.

From afar they say "Everything is alright", and off they go feeling themselves satisfied with what they saw.

I proceed now to lay before you few facts gathered from my experience.

To begin with- The inmates are not given hot water, but they get cold water shower – bath, and are confined every two hours. At night the noise is intolerable, recurring every two hours, especially of the peons and the *Halalcores*, [sweepers] who talk loudly. Though a surgeon is incharge who lives close by, he does not take the trouble to come and see the condition of the inmates.

As regards to medicine it is not properly given; whatever is indispensable it is never given.

The bedding is made of straw which is dangerous. Supposing someone uses a match it will ignite the bedding and with it other things, which will prove highly destructive.

The copper pots used for the water closet contain some disinfecting powder, which when for washing purposes, excites the parts of persons suffering from piles, as in my case, to which no heed is paid.

Would like to be furnished with a report in my case, when I left the Asylum, I was not given a certificate although I was asked for one as provided by the law.

I remained Sir,
Your most obedient Servant.
Sajan Curim[2]

---

[2] From Sajan Curim to the Secretary to the Government of Bombay, 16 October 1893, GoB, GD, 1893/75, MSA.

Glossary

A'rádhis Praying beggars (Hindu—from all caste groups)
Aatman The essence or spirit of Brahma (the creator in Hindu tradition) that inhabits in creation
Atharvan Sorcerer priest
Ayah Female attendant/wardress
Begar Unpaid forced labour
Bhagats Devotees
Bhámtas Also known as *Uchlias* (literally meaning 'lifters'); the *Gazetteer of the Bombay Presidency, Poona* accuses them of moving in groups to commit theft. It also notes that the *Bhámtas* 'occasionally suffer from spirit possession'.
Bhang A variation of hemp
Bháts A community of Maratha and Gujarati descent known to engage in different forms of manual labour. The *Gazetteer of the Bombay Presidency, Poona* labels them as 'hereditary beggars'.
Bhut Ghost
Brahmaraksasa Ghost of a Brahman who led an unholy life or a demon
Bundies Inner wear for upper body, similar to a vest
Chappals Slippers
Charas A variation of hemp
Chawl A type of housing unit in India used by the lower-middle or poor classes

© The Author(s) 2018
S. A. Pinto, *Lunatic Asylums in Colonial Bombay*,
Mental Health in Historical Perspective,
https://doi.org/10.1007/978-3-319-94244-5

Cholnas Type of short breeches
Choolies Plural form of choli, a blouse or bodice worn with a saree or lehanga
Cooly A workman, trained to deal with heavy loads
Cumblies/Kumblies Rough woollen blankets
Dhatus The seven tissues of the human body
Dhoties Garment which is worn on the lower body
Fakir Ascetic/Religious mendicant
Fenny Local alcoholic drink brewed from cashew
Gandharvas A Celestial being known to cause possession and ecstasy
Ganja A variation of Hemp
Geegras A type of skirt worn under a saree
Ghondalis A Hindu community known for performing the *ghondal* dance; the *Gazetteer* classifies them as a community of Hindu beggars
Ghury Clock
Hakim Muslim doctor of Unani
Kutcherry Office
Mali Gardener
Langorties Underwear for the lower body
Mofussil/Mufassal Areas outside the main urban centres of the Presidency
Pagal Khana Indian term for lunatic asylum
Pawrah/Pawada An agricultural hoe used in farming and construction
Perana A type of shirt
Picasa Demon
Pugdies/Pugris Plural form of *pugdi/pugri,* a turban/head gear
Raksasa Demon
Rupees (Rs.) Indian currency
Sadees Saree
Sadhu Ascetic/religious mendicant
Sudra A sacred muslin undershirt worn by the Parsis
Vaid/Vaidya/Vaidus Hindu doctor of Ayurveda or a physician
Yaksa Spirit or demi-god

BIBLIOGRAPHY

PRIMARY SOURCES

Maharashtra State Archives, Mumbai, India

Public Department Diaries (1793–1824)
Annual Report of the Colaba Lunatic Asylum
Dispatches from the PWD to the GoB
Letters from the Superintendent to the GoB
Lunacy Certificates

General Department Files (1825–1933)
Annual Report of the Asylums in the Bombay Presidency (1852–1871)
Asylum General Rules (Bombay Presidency)
Block Plans of the NMLA and Ratnagiri Lunatic Asylum
Circular to Magistrates, Bombay Presidency
Extracts from the Daily Register of Solitary Confinement
Extracts from the Reports of Visitors
Finance and Commerce Department Dispatches
GoB Memorandums
GoB Proceedings
GoB Resolutions
Letters from a patient to the GoB.

© The Author(s) 2018   217
S. A. Pinto, *Lunatic Asylums in Colonial Bombay*,
Mental Health in Historical Perspective,
https://doi.org/10.1007/978-3-319-94244-5

Letters from Asylum Staff to superintendents.
Letters from superintendents to the Civil Department
Letters from superintendents to the Judicial Department
Letters from superintendents to the Medical Board
Letters from the IMD to the Superintendent.
Letters from the Judicial Department to superintendents
Letters from the local community to the GoB
Letters from the Medical Board to the superintendents
Letters from the Superintendent to the IMD
Letters from the Survey Commissioner to the GoB
Lunacy Act XXXVI of 1858.
Lunacy Forms.
Map showing the location of the Colaba Lunatic Asylum
Medical Certificates issued to patients
Petitions/Letters to the Superintendent from families for the release of relatives
Rules for the Lunatic Asylums in the Bombay Presidency
Statements of Patients as Witnesses

REPORTS ON NATIVE NEWSPAPERS (1856–1909)

National Archives of India, New Delhi, India

Home Department Public Proceedings
Medical Proceedings, Home Department, Simla Records, GoI
Proceedings of the GoB

India Office Records, British Library, London, UK

Annual Report of the Bombay Lunatic Asylum, 31 March 1849, Board Collections, 1849–51
GoB, Board Collection
Letters dispatched to the GoB
Letters from Colney Hatch Lunatic Asylum to the GoB
Letters from the Penal Department to the GoI
Letters from the Superintendent to the GoB (Colaba Asylum)

National Library of Scotland, Scotland, UK. (Digital Resources)

Annual Administration and Progress Report on the Lunatic Asylums in the Bombay Presidency, 1873–1921

Annual Report on the Working of the Ranchi Indian Mental Hospital, Kanke in Bihar

Annual Reports on Mental Hospitals in the Bombay Presidency, 1922–1933.

Report of the Indian Hemp Drugs Commission, 1894–1895, Vol. 1–2

Heras Institute of Indian History and Culture, St Xavier's College, Mumbai, India

Triennial Report on the Civil Hospitals and Dispensaries of the Bombay Presidency (1923–1925)

Journals

British Journal of Psychiatry. http://bjp.rcpsych.org/content/by/year/

Indian Medical Gazette. https://archive.org/details/indianmedicalga00unkngoog

Medico -Chirurgical Review and Journal of Practical Medicine. https://books.google.co.nz/books?id=bxoUAAAAQAAJ&pg=PA397&lpg=PA397&dq=Dr+Ainslie+Whitelaw+Materia+Medica+of+Hindoostan&source=bl&ots=ywb9FPuzQy&sig=opwQPjOC1xmMPAJ7swJDUxO7vZM&hl=en&sa=X&ved=0ahUKEwjbs4Ot-NnQAhUDUbwKHaJjDVo4ChDoAQgrMAQ#v=onepage&q=Dr%20Ainslie%20Whitelaw%20Materia%20Medica%20of%20Hindoostan&f=false

The Monthly Review. https://books.google.co.nz/books?id=OA8oAAAAYAAJ&printsec=frontcover#v=onepage&q&f=false

Newspapers

Bombay Gazette
Indian Express
The Hindu
The Wall Street Journal

PUBLISHED PRIMARY SOURCES

Bartholomeo, Fra. 1800. *A Voyage to the East Indies*. Trans. William Johnson. London: J Davies.

Bernadotte, Lyon Isidore. 1921. *Medical Jurisprudence for India, with Illustrative Cases*. Vol. 7. Calcutta: Thacker and Spink.

Bowring, John, ed. 1843. *The Works of Jeremy Bentham*. Vol. 4. Edinburgh: William Tait.

Campbell, James, ed. 1879. *Gazetteer of the Bombay Presidency: Ahmedabad*. Vol. IV. Bombay: Government Central Press.

———. 1882. *Gazetteer of the Bombay Presidency: Thana*. Vol. XIII. Bombay: Government Central Press.

———. 1884. *Gazetteer of the Bombay Presidency: Belgaum District*. Bombay: Government Central Press.

———. 1885. *Gazetteers of the Bombay Presidency: Poona*. Vol. XVIII, Part 1. Bombay: Government Central Press.

———. 1886. *Gazetteer of the Bombay Presidency: Kolhapur District*. Vol. 24. Bombay: Government Central Press.

———. 1894. Notes on the Spirit Basis of Belief and Customs. *Indian Antiquary* 23: 374–384.

Conolly, John. 1847. *The Construction and Government of Lunatic Asylums as Hospitals for the Insanes*. London: John Church Hill.

———. 1856. *The Treatment of the Insane Without Mechanical Restraints*. London: Smith, Elder and Co.

Cox, Edmund. 1887. *A Short History of the Bombay Presidency*. Bombay: Thacker and Co.

Crawford, D.G. 1914. *A History of the Indian Medical Service, 1600–1913*. London: W Thacker and Co.

Dhunjibhoy, Jal Eduji. 1930. A Brief Resume of the Types of Insanity Commonly Met with in India, with a Full Description of the "Indian Hemp Insanity" Peculiar to the Country. *British Journal of Psychiatry* 76: 254–264.

Edwardes, S.M. 1909. *Gazetteer of Bombay City and Island*. Vol. 1. Bombay: Times Press.

———. 1912. *By-ways of Bombay*. Bombay: D.B. Taraporevala and Sons.

———. 1932. District Administration in Bombay 1858–1919. In *The Cambridge History of the British Empire, 1497–1858*, ed. H.D. Dodwell, vol. VI, 2nd ed., 58–74. London: Cambridge University Press.

Elliot, F.A.H., ed. 1883. *Gazetteer of the Bombay Presidency: Baroda*. Vol. VII, 619. Bombay: Government Central Press.

Ewens, George. 1903. An Account of a Race of Idiots Found in the Punjab, Commonly Known as "Shah Daula's Mice". *Indian Medical Gazette*, 38: 330–334. In *Disability Care and Education in 19th Century India: Dates, Places and*

Documentation with Some Additional Material on Mental Retardation and Physical Disabilities, Document Type: Information Analyses, ed. M. Miles. U.S. Department of Education, May 1997, 25–26.

Framjee, Dosabhoy. 1858. *The Parsees Their History, Manners, Customs and Religions.* Bombay/London: Smith Elder and Co.

Hughes, A.W. 1874. *A Gazetteer of the Province of Sindh.* London: George Bell and Sons.

Hunter, Wilson William. 1892. *Bombay 1885–1890: A Study in Indian Administration.* London/Bombay: H. Frowde/B.M. Malabari.

Hymns of the Atharva –Veda. 1895. Trans. Ralph T.H. Griffith. London: Luzac and Co.

Jehangir, Cowasji Jehangir. 1890. *Life of Sir Cowasjee Jehangir Readymoney, Kt., C.S.I., &c., &c.* London: London Stereoscopic and Photographic Company.

Johnson, William. 1866. *The Oriental Races and Tribes, Residents and Visitors of Bombay: A Series of Photographs with Letter-Press Descriptions.* Vol. 2. London: W.J. Johnson.

Lovett, Verney. 1932. The Development of the Services, 1858–1918. In *The Cambridge History of the British Empire, 1497–1858,* ed. H.D. Dodwell, vol. VI, 2nd ed., 357–376. London: Cambridge University Press.

Overbeck-Wright, A.W. 1912. *Mental Derangements in India: Its Symptoms and Treatment.* Calcutta/Simla: Thacker, Spink and Co.

———. 1921. *Lunacy in India.* London: Bailliere, Tindall and Cox.

Report of the Special Rapporteur on the Right of Everyone to the Enjoyment if the Highest Attainable Standard of Physical and Mental health, Human Rights Council, 28 March 2017, Thirty-Fifth Session, 6–23 June 2017.

Scholz, F. 1890. *Handbook of Mental Science.* Leipzig: Mayer.

Shaw, Jagoe W.S. 1932. Alienist Department of India. *British Journal of Psychiatry* 78: 331–341.

Sheppard, Samuel T. 1916. *The Byculla Club, 1833–1916: A History.* Bombay: Bennet, Coleman and Co.

———. 1917. *Bombay Place-Names and Street-Names: An Excursion into the By-Ways of the History of Bombay City.* Bombay: Times Press.

Simhaji, Bhagavat. 1896. *A Short History of Aryan Medical Science, 1865–1944.* London/New York: Macmillan and Co.

The Imperial Gazetteer of India: The Indian Empire, Administrative. Vol. IV. 1909. Oxford: Clarendon Press.

Wacha, Edulji Dinsha. 1910. *A Financial Chapter in the History of Bombay City.* Bombay: A.J. Combridge and Co.

Warnock, John. 1903. Insanity from Hasheesh. *British Journal of Psychiatry* 49: 96–110.

Whitelaw, Ainslie. 1813. *Materia Medica of Hindoostan, and Artisan's and Agriculturist's Nomenclature.* Madras: Government Press.

———. 1826. *Materia Indica; or, Some Account of Those Articles Which Are Employed by the Hindoos and Other Eastern nations, in Their Medicine, Arts, and Agriculture: Comprising also Formulae, with Practical Observations, Names of Diseases in Various Eastern Languages, and a Copious List of Oriental Books Immediately Connected with General Science, &c.* London: Longman, Rees, Orme, Brown and Green.

Williams, L.F. Rushbrook. 1924. *India in 1923–24.* Calcutta: Government of India, Central Publication Branch.

WEBSITES

http://www.ohchr.org/en/NewsEvents/Pages/DisplayNews.aspx?News ID=21689&LangID=E. Accessed 15 Aug 2017.

https://www.britannica.com/biography/Robert-Napier-1st-Baron-Napier. Accessed 5 Oct 2016.

Mirabai -54 Poems-, Classic Poetry Series. 2012. http://www.poemhunter. com/i/ebooks/pdf/mirabai_2012_7.pdf. Accessed 14 July 2015.

National Mental Health Program. 1982. http://mohfw.nic.in/WriteReadData/ 1892s/9903463892NMHP%20detail.pdf. Accessed 21 Oct 2016.

Tissues/ Dhatus. https://www.ayurvedacollege.com/articles/drhalpern/the-seven-dhatus-tissues-ayurveda. Accessed 8 Oct 2016.

SECONDARY SOURCES

Alyonaa, Baltabayeva, Tursunb Gabitov, Akmarala Maldubek, and Sairab Shamakhay. 2016. Spiritual Understanding of Human Rights in Muslim Culture (The Problem of "Ruh" – "Spirit"). *Procedia – Social and Behavioural Sciences,* 217: 712–718.

Arnold, David. 1993. *Colonizing the Body: State Medicine and Epidemic Disease in Nineteenth-Century India.* Berkley: University of California Press.

———. 1994. Public Health and Public Power: Medicine and Hegemony in Colonial India. In *Contesting Colonial Hegemony: State and Society in Africa and India,* ed. Daglar Engles and Shula Marks, 131–151. London/New York: British Academic Press.

Bala, Poonam. 2012. "Nationalizing" Medicine: The Changing Paradigm of Ayurveda in British India. In *Contesting Colonial Authority: Medicine and Indigenous Responses in Nineteenth and Twentieth–Century India,* ed. Poonam Bala, 1–12. Lanham/Boulder/New York/Toronto/Plymouth: Lexington Books.

Balan, Sergiu. 2010. Foucault's View on Power Relations. *Cogito: Multidisciplinary Research Journal* 2 (2): 37–42.

Bartlett, Peter. 2000. Structures of Confinement in 19th-Century Asylums. *International Journal of Law and Psychiatry* 23 (1): 1–13.

Bayly, C.A. 1996. *Empire and Information: Intelligence Gathering and Social Communication in India, 1780–1870.* New York: Cambridge University Press.

Beck, Brenda E.F. 1969. Colour and Heat in South Indian Ritual. *Man*, New Series, 4 (4): 553–572.

Buckingham, Jane. 2002. *Leprosy in Colonial South India Medicine and Confinement.* Basingstoke: Palgrave Macmillan.

Busfield, Joan. 1994. The Female Malady? Men, Women and Madness in Nineteenth-Century Britain. *Sociology* 28 (1): 259–277.

Chakravarti, Uma. 1995. Ageing, Gender Caste and Labour: Ideological and Material Structure of Widowhood. *Economic and Political Weekly* 30 (36): 2248–2256.

Chaudhuri, Nirad. 1976. *Culture in the Vanity Bag.* Bombay: Jaico.

Cohn, Bernard. 1996. *Colonialism and Its Forms of Knowledge.* Princeton: Princeton University Press.

Coleborne, Catharine. 2010. *Madness in the Family: Insanity and Institutions in the Australasian Colonial World, 1860–1914.* Basingstoke: Palgrave Macmillan.

Cook, Ian, and Michelle Harrison. 2003. Cross Over Food: Rematerializing Postcolonial Geographies. *Transactions of the Institute of British Geographers* 28: 296–317.

Deacon, Harriet. 2003. Insanity, Institutions and Society: the Case of the Robben Island Lunatic Asylum, 1846–1910. In *The Confinement of the Insane: International Perspectives, 1800–1965*, ed. Roy Porter and David Wright, 20–53. New York: Cambridge University Press.

Denault, Leigh. 2009. Partition and the Joint Family in the Nineteenth–Century North India. *The Indian Economic and Social History Review* 46 (1): 27–55.

Dietler, Michael. 2007. Culinary Encounters: Food, Identity and Colonialism. In *The Archaeology of Food and Identity*, ed. Katheryn C. Twiss, 218–242. Carbondale: Southern Illinois University Press.

Dirks, Nicholas. 1996. Foreward. In *Colonialism and Its Forms of Knowledge*, ed. Bernard Cohn, ix–xvii. Princeton: Princeton University Press.

———. 2001. *Castes of Mind: Colonialism and the Making of Modern India.* Princeton: Princeton University Press.

Doerner, Klaus. 1981. *Madmen and the Bourgeoisie: A Social History of Insanity and Psychiatry.* Oxford: Blackwell Publishers.

Dotson, Kirstie. 2011. Tracking Epistemic Violence, Tracking Practices of Silences. *Hypatia* 26 (2): 236–257.

Duran, Eduardo. 2006. *Healing the Soul Wound: Counselling with American Indian and Other Native People.* New York: Teachers College Press.

Dzuvichu, L. 2014. Empire on Their Backs: Coolies in the Eastern Borderland of the British Raj. *International Review of Social Histroy* 59 (Special Issue): 89–112.

Edgar, R., and H. Sapire. 2000. *African Apocalypse: The Story of Nontetha Nkwenkwe, a Twentieth- Century South African Prophet.* Johannesburg: Witwatersrand University Press.

Elankumaran, S. 2004. Personality, Organizational Climate and Job Involvement: An Empirical Study. *Journal of Human Values* 10 (2): 117–130.

Ernst, Waltraud. 1991a. Racial, Social and Cultural Factors in the Development of a Colonial Institution: The Bombay Lunatic Asylum (1670–1858). *Internationales Asienforum* 22 (3–4): 61–80.

———. 1991b. Out of Sight and Out of Mind: Insanity in Early 19th Century British India. In *Insanity, Institutions and Society, 1800–1914,* Studies in the Social History of Medicine, ed. Joseph Melling and Bill Forsythe, 245–268. London/New York: Routledge.

———. 1996. European Madness and Gender in Nineteenth-Century British India. *Social History of Medicine* 9 (3): 357–382.

———. 1997. Idioms of Madness and Colonial Boundaries: The Case of the European and "Native" Mentally Ill in Early Nineteenth-Century British India. *Comparative Studies in Society and History* 39 (01): 153–181.

———. 1999. Colonial Policies, Racial Politics and the Development of Psychiatric Institutions in the Early Nineteenth-Century British India. In *Race, Science and Medicine, 1700–1960,* ed. Waltraud Ernst and Bernard Harris. London: Routledge, Taylor and Francis Group.

———. 2006. Medical/Colonial Power-Lunatic Asylum in Bengal, c. 1800-1900. *Journal of Asian History* 40 (1): 49–79.

———. 2007. Madness and Colonial Spaces in British India. In *Madness, Architecture and the Built Environment: Psychiatric Spaces in Historical Context,* ed. Leslie Topp, James Moran, and Jonathan Andrews, 215–238. New York/London: Routledge.

———. 2010. *Mad Tales from the Raj: Colonial Psychiatry in South Asia, 1800–58.* New York: Anthem Press.

———. 2012. The Indianization of Colonial Medicine: The Case of Psychiatry in the Early–Twentieth Century British India. *NTM International Journal of History & Ethics of Natural Sciences, Technology and Medicine* 20: 61–89.

———. 2013. *Colonialism and Transnational Psychiatry: The Development of an Indian Mental Hospital in British India, 1925–1930.* London/New York: Anthem Press.

Fennelly, Katherine. 2014. Out of Sound, Out of Mind: Noise Control in Nineteenth-Century Lunatic Asylums in England and Ireland. *World Archaeology* 46 (3): 416–430.

Finnane, Mark. 1981. *Insanity and the Insane in Post-Famine Ireland*. Totowa: Barnes and Noble.

———. 1985. Asylums, Families and the State. *History Workshop Journal* 20: 134–148.

Fischer-Tiné, Harald. 2005. Britain's Other Civilizing Mission: Class Prejudice, European 'loaferism' and the Workhouse-System in Colonial India. *The Indian Economic and Social History Review* 42 (3): 295–338.

Foucault, Michel. 1977. *Discipline and Punish: The Birth of the Prison*. Trans. Alan Sheridan. New York: Random House.

———. 1980. *Power/Knowledge: Selected Interviews and Other Writings, 1972–1977*. New York: Pantheon.

———. 2003. *Madness and Civilization: A History of Insanity in the Age of Reason*. Trans. Richard Howard. New York: Vintage Books.

———. 2006. *History of Madness*. Trans. Jonathan Murphy and Jean Khalfa. London: Routledge Taylor and Francis Group.

Garton, Stephen. 1988. *Medicine and Madness: a Social History of Insanity in New South Wales, 1880–1940*. Kensington: New South Wales University Press.

Goffman, Erving. 1961. *Asylums: Essays on the Social Situation of Mental Patients and Other Inmates*. New York: Anchor Books.

Gramsci, Antonio. 1971. *Selections from Prison Notebooks*. New York: International Publishers.

Green, Nile. 2014. Breaking the Begging Bowl: Morals, Drugs, and Madness in the Fate of the Muslim Faqir. *South Asian History and Culture* 5 (2): 226–245.

Guha, Ranajit. 1997. *Dominance Without Hegemony: History and Power in Colonial India*. Cambridge, MA/London: Harvard University Press.

Gupta, Aakhil. 1995. Blurred Boundaries: The Discourse of Corruption, the Culture of Politics, and the Imagines State. *American Ethnologist* 22 (2): 375–402.

Harrison, Mark. 1994. *Public Health in British India: Anglo Indian Preventive Medicine, 1859–1914*. Melbourne: Cambridge University Press.

Haynes, D.E. 1987. From Tribute to Philanthropy: The Politics of Gift Giving in a Western Indian City. *The Journal of Asian Studies* 46 (2): 339–360.

Haynes, Doughlas, and Gyan Prakash, eds. 1991. *Resistance and Everyday Social Relations in South Asia*. Delhi: Oxford University Press.

Headrick, Daniel. 1981. *The Tools of Empire: Technology and European Imperialism in the Nineteenth Century*. New York: Oxford University Press.

Hofstede, Geert. 1991. *Culture and Organizations: Software of the Mind*. London: McGraw Hill.

Jain, Sanjeev. 2003. Psychiatry and Confinement in India. In *The Confinement of the Insane: International Perspectives, 1800–1965*, ed. Roy Porter and David Wright, 273–298. New York: Cambridge University Press.

Joseph, M.T. 2007. Migration and Identity Formation: A Case Study of Dalit Assertion in Aurangabad, Maharashtra. In *Migration and Mission in India*, ed. Joseph Jose and L. Stanislaus, 95–124. New Delhi: ISPCK.

Kakar, Sudhir. 1982. *Shamans, Mystics and Doctors*. Chicago: The University of Chicago Press.

Kalant, Oriana. 1972. Report of the Indian Hemp Drugs Commission, 1893–94: A Critical Review. *The International Journal of the Addictions* 7 (1): 77–96.

Kalpagam, U. 2002. Colonial Governmentality and the Public Sphere in India. *Journal of Historical Sociology* 15 (1): 35–58.

Kavadi, Shirish. 2015. Philanthropy, Medicine and Health in Colonial India. In *Encyclopaedia of the History of Science, Technology, and Medicine in Colonial India*, 1–9. Netherlands: Springer.

Kerr, Ian J. 2003. Representation and Representations of Railways of Colonial and Post-Colonial South Asia. *Modern Asian Studies* 37 (2): 287–326.

Khalid, Amna. 2009. Subordinate Negotiations; Indigenous Staff, the Colonial State and Public Health. In *The Social History of Health and Medicine in Colonial India*, ed. Biswamoy Pati and Mark Harrison, 45–73. New York: Routledge.

Kosambi, Meera. 1996. Konkan Ports and European Dominance: An Urban Perspective. In *Mediaeval Deccan History: Commemoration Volume in Honour of Purshottam Mahadeo Joshi*, ed. A.R. Kulkarni, M.A. Nayeem, and T.R. de Souza, 108–123. Bombay: Popular Prakashan.

Kulke, Eckehard. 1974. *The Parsees in India: A Minority as Agent of Social Change*. Munchen: Weltforum Verlag.

Kumar, Anil. 1998. *Medicine and the Raj: British Medical Policy in India, 1835–1911*. New Delhi: Altamira Press.

Lamb, Sarah. 1999. Aging, Gender and Widowhood: Perspectives from Rural West Bengal. *Contributions to Indian Sociology* 33 (3): 541–570.

Leckie, Jacqueline. 2004. Modernity and Management of Madness in Colonial Fiji. *Paideuma* 50: 251–274.

Leong–Salobir, Cecelia. 2011. *Food Culture in Colonial Asia: A Taste of Empire*. London/New York: Routledge.

Levine, Philippa. 2008. States of Undress: Nakedness and the Colonial Imagination. *Victorian Studies* 50 (2): 189–219.

———. 2013. Naked Truths: Bodies, Knowledge, and the Erotics of Colonial Power. *Journal of British Studies* 52 (1): 5–25.

Mackinnon, Dolly. 2003. Hearing Madness the Soundscape of the Asylum. In *Madness in Australia: Histories, Heritage and the Asylum*, ed. Catharine Coleborne and Dolly Mackinnon, 73–82. Queensland: Queensland University Press.

———. 2003. 'Jolly and Fond of Singing': The Gendered Nature of Musical Entertainment in Queensland Mental Institutions, c1870–1937. In *Madness in Australia*, ed. Catharine Coleborne and Dolly Mackinnon, 157–168. Queensland: Queensland University Press.

Malcolm, Elizabeth. 2003. "Ireland's Crowded Madhouses": The Institutional Confinement of the Insane in Nineteenth- and Twentieth-Century Ireland. In *The Confinement of the Insane: International Perspectives, 1800–1965*, ed. Roy Porter and David Wright, 315–333. New York: Cambridge University Press.

Mandelbaum, David. 1970. *Society in India*. Berkley: University of California Press.

Mann, Michael. 2003. Torchbearers Upon the Path of Progress: Britain's Ideology of Moral and Material Progress in India. In *Colonialism as Civilising Mission*, ed. Harald Fischer-Tiné and Michael Mann. London: Anthem Press.

Marfatia, J.A. 1961. Welfare of the Mentally Handicapped. In *History and Philosophy Social Work in India*, ed. A.R. Wadia, 361–382. Bombay: Allied Publishers.

McCulloh, Jock. 1995. *Colonial Psychiatry and 'The African Mind'*. Cambridge: Cambridge University Press.

Mills, James. 2000. *Madness, Cannabis and Colonialism: The 'Native-Only' Lunatic Asylums of British India, 1857–1900*. Basingstoke: Macmillan Press Limited.

———. 2001. The History of Modern Psychiatry in India, 1858–1947. *History of Psychiatry* 12: 431–458.

———. 2003. "More Important to Civilise than Subdue"? Lunatic Asylums, Psychiatric Practice and Fantasies of the "Civilising Mission" in British India 1858—1900. In *Colonialism as Civilising Mission*, ed. Harald Fischer-Tiné and Michael Mann, 171–182. London: Anthem Press.

———. 2009. Psychiatry on Edge? Vagrants, Families, and Colonial Asylums in India, 1857–1900. In *Fringes of Empire*, ed. Sameetah Agha and Elizabeth Kolsky, 188–206. New Delhi: Oxford University Press.

Moran, James. 2001. *Committed to the State Asylum: Insanity and Society in Nineteenth-Century Quebec and Ontario*. Montreal/Kingston/London/Ithaca: McGill-Queen's University Press.

Mukherjee, Dyutimoy. 2008. Laws for Beggars, Justice for Whom: A Critical Review of the Bombay Prevention of Begging Act 1959. *The International Journal of Human Rights* 12 (2): 279–288.

Mushtaq, Muhammad Umair. 2009. Public Health in British India: A Brief Account of the History of Medical Services and Disease Prevention in Colonial India'. *Indian Journal Community Med* 34 (1): 6–14.

Nandy, Ashish. 1983. *The Intimate Enemy: Loss and Recovery of Self Under Colonialism*. Delhi: Oxford University Press.

Narayan, Govind. 2009. *Mumbai: An Urban Biography from 1863*. Trans. Murali Ranganathan. New York: Anthem Press.

Neaman, Judith. 1975. *Suggestions of the Devil: The Origins of Madness*. New York: Anchor Press.

Nigam, Sanjay. 1990. Disciplining and Policing the "Criminals by Birth", Part 1: The Making of a Colonial Stereotype—The Criminal Tribes and Castes of North India. *The Indian Economic and Social History Review* 27 (2): 131–164.

Oursel, Masson, Grabowska Paul De Willman, Stern Helena. 1951. *Ancient India and Indian Civilization*. Trans. M.R. Dobie. London: Kegan Paul, Trench, Trubner & Co.

Owen, Margaret. 1996. *A World of Widows*. London: Zed Books.

Pandey, Gyanendra. 2014. Unarchived Histories: The "Mad" and the "Trifling". In *Unarchived Histories: The "Mad" and the "Trifling" in the Colonial and Postcolonial World*, ed. Gyanendra Pandey, 1–20. London/New York: Routledge.

Parle, Julie. 2003. Witchcraft or Madness? The Amandiki of Zululand, 1894–1914. *Journal of Southern African Studies* 29 (1): 105–132.

———. 2004. *States of Mind: Mental Illness and the Quest for Mental Health in Natal and Zululand, 1868–1918*. PhD Thesis, University of KwaZulu-Natal.

Parry-Jones, William Ll. 1972. *The Trade in Lunacy: A Study of Private Madhouses in England in the Eighteenth and Nineteenth Centuries*. London: Routledge and Keenan Paul.

Piddock, Susan. 2007. *A Space of Their Own: The Archaeology of Nineteenth-Century Lunatic Asylums in Britain, South Australia and Tasmania*. New York: Springer.

Pietikainen, Petteri. 2015. *Madness: A History*. London/New York: Routledge Taylor and Francis Group.

Porter, Roy. 1987. *Mind–Forg'd Menacles: A History of Madness in England from Restoration to the Regency*. London: Althone Press.

———. 2003. Introduction. In *The Confinement of the Insane: International Perspectives, 1800–1965*, ed. Roy Porter and David Wright. New York: Cambridge University Press.

Prakash, Gyan. 1999. *Another Reason: Science and the Imagination of Modern India*. Princeton: Princeton University Press.

Rajpal, Shilpi. 2015a. Colonial Psychiatry in Mid-Nineteenth Century India: The James Clark Enquiry. *South Asia Research* 35 (1): 61–80.

———. 2015b. Quotidian Madness: Time, Management and Asylums in Colonial North India. *Studies in History* 31 (2): 206–234.

Ramanna, Mridula. 2001. Gauging Indian Responses to Western Medicine: Hospitals and Dispensaries, Bombay Presidency, 1900–1920. In *Disease and Medicine in India: A Historical Review*, ed. Deepak Kumar, 233–248. New Delhi: Tulika Books.

———. 2002. *Western Medicine and Public Health in Colonial Bombay, 1845–1895*. New Delhi: Orient Longman.

Rao, Ursula. 2010. *News as Culture: Journalistic Practices and the Remaking of Indian Leadership Traditions*. New York: Berghahn Books.

Ray, Avishek. 2014. *Archaeology of Vagabondage: South Asia's Colonial Encounter.* PhD Thesis, Trent University.

Reaume, Geoffery. 2006. Insane Asylum Inmates' Labour in Ontario, 1841–1900. In *Mental Health and Canadian Society,* ed. James Moran and David Wright, 69–96. Montreal/Kingston/London/Ithaca: McGill-Queen's University Press.

Richmond, Vivienne. 2013. *Clothing the Poor in Nineteenth-Century England.* Cambridge: Cambridge University Press.

Roman, et al. 2009. No Time for Nostalgia!: Asylum-making, Medicalized Colonialism in British Columbia (1859–97) and Artistic Praxis for Social Transformation. *International Journal of Qualitative Studies in Education* 22 (1): 17–63.

Sadowsky, Jonathan. 1997. Psychiatry and Colonial Ideology in Nigeria. *Bulletin of the History of Medicine* 71 (1): 94–111.

———. 1999. *Imperial Bedlam: Institutions of Madness in Colonial Southwest Nigeria.* Berkeley: University of California Press.

———. 2003. Confinement and Colonialism in Nigeria. In *The Confinement of the Insane: International Perspectives, 1800–1965,* ed. Roy Porter and David Wright, 299–314. New York: Cambridge University Press.

Said, Edward. 1979. *Orientalism.* New York: Vintage.

Scott, James. 1985. *Weapons of the Weak: Everyday Forms of Peasant Resistance.* New Haven: Yale University Press.

Scull, Andrew. 1975. From Madness to Mental Illness: Medical Men as Moral Entrepreneurs. *European Journal of Sociology* 16 (2): 218–261.

———. 1979. *Museums of Madness: The Social Organization of Insanity in Nineteenth-Century England.* London: Trinity Press.

———. 1981a. *Madhouses, Mad-doctors, and Madmen: The Social History of Psychiatry in the Victorian Era.* Philadelphia: University of Pennsylvania Press.

———. 1981b. Discovery of the Asylum Revisited: Lunacy Reform in the New American Republic. In *Madhouses, Mad-Doctors, and Madmen,* ed. Andrew Scull, 144–165. London: Athlone Press.

———. 2015. *Madness in Civilization: A Cultural History of Insanity, from the Bible to Freud, from the Madhouse to Modern Medicine.* Princeton/Oxford: Princeton University Press.

Sen, Samita. 1999. *Women and Labour in Late Colonial India: The Bengal Jute Industry.* Cambridge: Cambridge University Press.

Sen, Satadru. 2002. The Savage Family: Colonialism and Female Infanticide in Nineteenth-Century India. *Journal of Women's History* 14 (3): 53–79.

Shakespear, John. 2002. *John Shakespears's Dictionary: Urdu-English and English to Urdu.* Lahore: Sang-e-Meel.

Sharma, S. 1990. *Mental Hospitals in India.* New Delhi: Director General of Health Services.

Sharma, S., and L.P. Varma. 1984. History of Mental Hospitals in the Indian Subcontinent. *Indian Journal of Psychiatry* 26 (4): 295–300.

Shekhawat, R. 2012. Black Sufis: Preserving the Siddi's and Its Age-old Culture in India, 4th Indian Hospitality Congress – India, Paper Presentation.

Showalter, Elaine. 1985. *The Female Malady*. New York: Pantheon Books.

Siber, Mouloud, and Bouteldja Riche. 2013. The Aesthetic of Natives' Dress and Undress: Colonial Stereotype and Mimicry in Paul Gauguin's and William Somerset Maugham's Cultural Forms. *Linguistic Practices* 19: 27–48.

Siebenga, Rianne. 2012. Colonial India's "Fanatical Fakirs" and Their Popular Representations. *History and Anthropology* 23 (4): 445–466.

Singh, Hulas. 2016. *Rise of Reason: Intellectual History of 19th-Century Maharashtra*. New York: Routledge.

Singhal, K.C., and Roshan Gupta. 2003. *The Ancient History of India, Vedic Period: A New Interpretation*. New Delhi: Atlantic Publishers and Distributors.

Sinha, J.B.P. 2014. *Psycho-Social Analysis of the Indian Mindset*. New Delhi/New York/Heidelberg/Dordrecht: Springer.

Skultans, Vieda. 1975. *Madness and Morals: Ideas on Insanity in the Nineteenth Century*. London: Routledge and Kegan Paul.

Slocum, Rachel. 2011. Race in the Study of Food. *Progress in Human Geography* 35 (3): 303–327.

Smith, Leonard. 1999. *Cure, Comfort and Safe Custody*. London/New York: Leicester University Press.

Smith, Cathy. 2006. Family, Community and the Victorian Asylum: A Case Study of the Northampton General Lunatic Asylum and Its Pauper Lunatics. *Family & Community History* 2 (2): 109–124.

Smith, Leonard. 2014. *Insanity, Race and Colonialism: Managing Mental Disorder in the Post-Emancipation British Caribbean, 1838–1914*. London: Palgrave Macmillan.

Spivak, G.C. 1988. Can the Subaltern Speak? In *Marxism and Interpretation of Culture*, ed. C. Nelson and L. Grossberg, 271–313. Chicago: University of Illinois Press.

Swartz, Sally. 1995. The Black Insane in Cape, 1891–1920. *Journal of Southern African Studies* 21 (3): 399–415.

———. 1999. Lost Lives: Gender, History and Mental Illness in the Cape. *Feminism and Psychology* 9 (2): 152–158.

———. 2010. The Regulation of British Colonial Lunatic Asylums and the Origins of Colonial Psychatry, 1860–1864. *American Psychological Association* 13 (2): 160–177.

Tarlo, Emma. 1996. *Clothing Matters: Dress and Identity in India*. Chicago: University of Chicago Press.

Tennant, Margaret. 1989. *Paupers and Providers: Charitable Aid in New Zealand*. Wellington: Allen and Unwin/Historical Branch.

Van Deth, Ron, and Walter Vandereychken. 2000. Food Refusal and Insanity: Sitophobia and Anorexia Nervosa in Victorian Asylums. *International Journal of Eating Disorders* 27 (4): 390–404.

Van Gabriel, Loon, ed. 2002. *Charakha Samhita: Handbook on Ayurveda*. Vol. II. New Delhi: Chaukhambha Orientalia Publishers.

Vaughan, Megan. 1991. *Curing their Ills: Colonial Power and African Illness*. Stanford: Stanford University Press.

Weiberger-Thomas, Catherine. 1999. *Ashes of Immortality: Widow Burining in India*. Trans. Jeffrey Mehlman and David Gordon White. Chicago: University of Chicago Press.

Weir, Christine. 2014. "We Visit the Colo Towns...When It Is Safe to Go": Indigenous Adoption of Methodist Christianity in the Wainibuka and Wainimala Valleys, Fiji, in the 1870s. *The Journal of Pacific History* 49 (2): 129–150.

Weiss, Mitchell. 1983. The Treatment of Insane Patients in India in the Lunatic Asylums of the Nineteenth Century. *Indian Journal of Psychiatry* 25 (4): 312–316.

Werner, Karel. 1988. Indian Concepts of Human Personality in Relation to the Doctrine of the Soul. *The Journal of the Royal Asiatic Society of Great Britain and Ireland* 1 (1): 73–97.

White, Richard. 1991. *The Middle Ground: Indians, Empires, and Republics in the Great Lakes Region, 1650–1815*. Cambridge: Cambridge University Press.

Williams, Monier M. 2005. *A Sanskrit -English Dictionary*. Delhi: Motilala Banarassidas Publishers.

Witzel, Michael. 1995. Early Sanskritization: Origins and Development of the Kuru State. *Electronic Journal of Vedic Studies (EJVS)* 1 (4): 27–52.

Wright, David. 1997. Getting Out of the Asylum: Understanding the Confinement of the Insane in the Nineteenth Century. *Social History of Medicine* 10 (1): 137–155.

———. 2000. Learning Disability and the New Poor Law in England, 1834–1867. *Disability and Society* 15 (5): 731–745.

Wright, David, Laurie Jacklin, and Tom Themeles. 2013. Dying to Get Out of the Asylum: Mortality and Madness in Four Mental Hospitals in Victorian Canada, c. 1841–1891. *Bulletin of the History of Medicine* 87 (4): 591–621.

PhD Thesis

Bhattacharyya, Anouska. 2013. *Indian Insanes, Lunacy in the "Native" Asylums of Colonial India, 1858–1912*. Ph.D Thesis, Harvard University.

Kapila, Shruti. 2002. *The Making of Colonial Psychiatry, Bombay Presidency, 1849–1940*. Ph.D Thesis, School of Oriental and African Studies, University of London.

Mills, James. 1997. *The Lunatic Asylum in British India, 1857 to 1880: Colonialism, Medicine and Power*. Ph.D Thesis, The University of Edinburgh.

INDEX[1]

[1] Note: Page numbers followed by 'n' refer to notes.

© The Author(s) 2018

S. A. Pinto, *Lunatic Asylums in Colonial Bombay*,
Mental Health in Historical Perspective,
https://doi.org/10.1007/978-3-319-94244-5

233

INDEX 241